The BIG BOOK of
GLUTEN-FREE COOKING

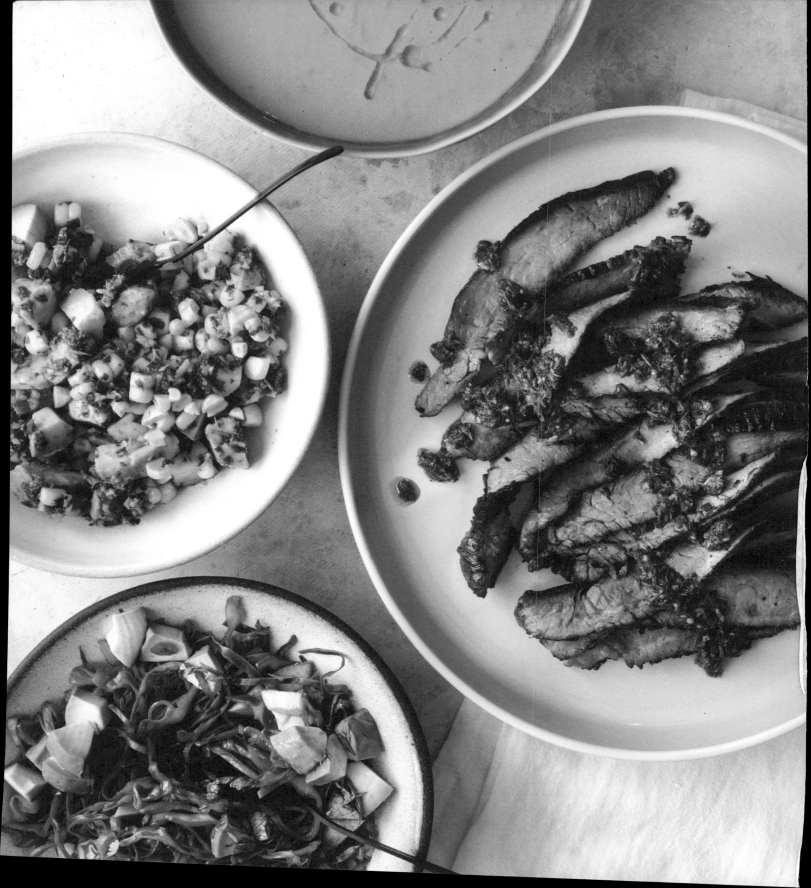

The BIG BOOK of GLUTEN-FREE COOKING

Delicious Meals, Breads, and Sweets
for a Happy, Healthy Gluten-Free Life

GIGI STEWART, B.S., M.A.

ROCKRIDGE
PRESS

For general information on our other products and services or to obtain technical support, please contact our Customer Care Department within the U.S. at (866) 744-2665, or outside the U.S. at (510) 253-0500.

Rockridge Press publishes its books in a variety of electronic and print formats. Some content that appears in print may not be available in electronic books, and vice versa.

TRADEMARKS: Rockridge Press and the Rockridge Press logo are trademarks or registered trademarks of Callisto Media Inc. and/or its affiliates, in the United States and other countries, and may not be used without written permission. All other trademarks are the property of their respective owners. Rockridge Press is not associated with any product or vendor mentioned in this book.

Cover Designer: William D. Mack
Interior Designer: Meg Woodcheke
Editor: Stacy Wagner-Kinnear
Production Editor: Erum Khan
Photography © Nadine Greeff except Hélène Dujardin/Food styling by Lisa Rovick, p. 28, 63, 150, 190, cover (pizza).

ISBN: Print 978-1-62315-983-2 | eBook 978-1-62315-984-9

Printed in canada

For Gracie

Contents

Introduction

Supermarket visits don't typically serve up standout moments. But there's one trip I'll never forget. It was October 26, 2007. I'd stopped in a local market to pick up some last-minute items for Halloween. Standing in the condiment aisle, I thumbed through my phone's contacts list for a friend's number. You could say I needed a lifeline. When the familiar voice answered, I skipped the greeting and asked anxiously, "Is ketchup gluten-free?"

That was three days after my celiac disease diagnosis, and I was clueless about gluten. At the time, information on the disease was scarce. "Gluten-free" was not a household term, but it quickly became one for my family. After 25 years of chronic pain, my diagnosis was a relief. I felt grateful to have a name for what had caused my health issues. Lacking the knowledge of exactly what I could eat, I was happy to have a simple meal of grilled steak, baked potato, and plain salad those first few days. Waking up every morning pain-free was worth it!

But as time passes, we need more than the same basic meal each day. We need to eat with the family, enjoy backyard barbecues, and join in on celebrations and holiday meals with ease. It can be as simple as ketchup on our fries or as complicated as a birthday layer cake. The key to mastering gluten-free living is knowing which foods to eat, which to avoid, and how to recreate our favorites so we aren't left feeling deprived.

Thinking back to that day in the supermarket is a grounding moment. It helps me remember that this gluten-free life can be hard. In the case of celiac disease, the dietary change must be immediate. There is no opportunity to ease into this new way of eating. For most people, as it was for me, the learning curve is steep and overwhelming. We quickly realize there is much more to living gluten-free than swapping regular foods for gluten-free versions. The availability of those products is not a guarantee that they taste good or are good for our health. So many differing opinions about which products are best only add to the confusion.

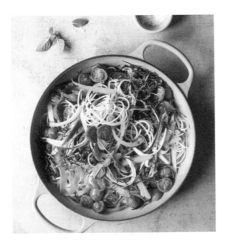
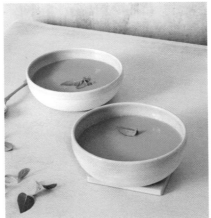
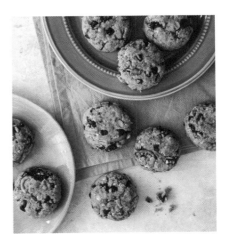

I've written *The Big Book of Gluten-Free Cooking* to end the confusion and make gluten-free living less overwhelming and, dare I say, enjoyable! My approach to gluten-free living is to keep it simple, affordable, nutritious, and fun. Like a lot of you, I have a family to feed, and I don't have time to prepare separate meals. That means the gluten-free dishes I serve must meet everyone's expectations. And regardless of what others say, you don't need a stack of specialty cookbooks or a culinary degree to make satisfying gluten-free food that no one will ever guess is gluten-free. You just need this book.

Here, you have dozens of recipes that happen to be naturally gluten-free, as well as dozens more I created to mimic the gluten-filled foods we all love and miss, like soft flour tortillas, sliceable sandwich bread, delicate yellow sheet cake, and authentic pizza crust. Yes, really!

Because other food allergies and intolerances often go along with celiac disease and gluten sensitivity, every recipe in this book is also completely free from soy, peanuts, and tree nuts. Nearly all recipes are dairy-free or offer a viable dairy-free option, and many are egg-free, too. You'll find variations and tips along the way to help you keep meals fresh and exciting year-round. These recipes are designed to support you in embracing the dietary changes you face, bring joy to your table, and change everyone's mind about gluten-free food.

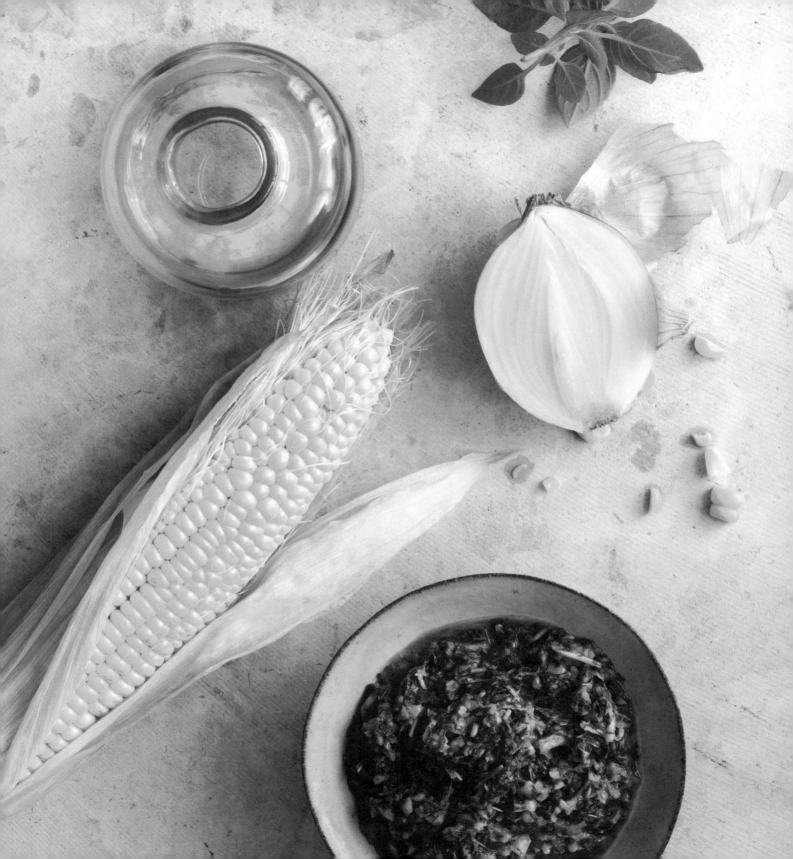

CHAPTER 1

Goodbye, Gluten
Hello, Health

Food is about so much more than keeping our bodies going. Food is connected to family, memories, and pleasure. With this in mind, saying goodbye to gluten can be downright depressing. But take heart. Your days of enjoying backyard barbecues and birthday party cupcakes are not over. We all deserve to eat well, just as much as we did before we had to, or decided to, give up gluten. With time, solid information, a bit of planning, and a slight adjustment in perspective, anyone can master gluten-free living and find joy in mealtime again.

Gluten in Brief

I'm sure you didn't give gluten much thought until you had to stop eating it—I certainly didn't. Whether I knew it or not, I depended on gluten, which I learned is a specific protein in grains like wheat, barley, and rye. It gives a New York–style bagel its chew, it makes cake layers so light and delicate we want to weep while eating them, and it is responsible for keeping muffins moist for days. It may surprise you to learn that gluten makes frequent appearances in other foods, too. From canned soups to yogurt to soy sauce, gluten flaunts its binding ability everywhere.

In reality, no one is able to digest gluten. That's not a problem for most people, but if you're one of the "chosen" with celiac disease or gluten sensitivity, your body made the decision that gluten must go in order for you to live a healthy life. With celiac disease, the body recognizes gluten as a foreign invader and mounts an immune response that destroys the lining of your small intestine. People with gluten sensitivity do not suffer gut damage, but they do experience some of the more than 300 symptoms associated with celiac disease. There are other diseases, like autoimmune thyroid disease, type 1 diabetes, and multiple sclerosis, that, while not directly caused by eating gluten, benefit from a gluten-free diet.

Even if a person eats gluten their entire life without apparent issues, one day symptoms can hit. That's when you find yourself sitting in a doctor's office being told you can't eat cookies or hamburger buns and that you won't be washing down pizza with a cold beer anymore. Unfortunately, when you are faced with eliminating gluten, friends and family members may decide you made up a "food allergy" for attention. You and I know this is ridiculous, but it's a real issue for many of us. It's not easy, but let them be. Our primary goal is your health.

The Joys of Getting Gluten Gone

Anything new can make us feel uncertain at first, but soon, living gluten-free will become second nature. Here are five benefits of giving up gluten:

1. Health mysteries are solved. With celiac disease, gluten sensitivity, or another gluten-related health diagnosis, confirmation of what is wrong and learning how to fix it comes as a huge relief.

2. Nutrients from foods you eat are absorbed. Healing your digestive system with a gluten-free diet means you reap the health benefits of the nutrients you consume. This gives your body what it needs to function properly.

3. Meals made at home bring a double bonus. The challenge of dining out gluten-free may seem like a drawback, but it can be a bonus. People who cook at home tend to be healthier, and it's healthier for your budget, too.

4. Foods you weren't aware of become new favorites. A gluten-free diet turns what we eat upside down. In some ways, that's great news. Delicious foods you might never have tried otherwise suddenly end up on your plate. Gluten-free whole grains like quinoa, amaranth, and teff add variety to meals. Exploring new fruits and vegetables and cooking with alternative flours can lead you on an exciting culinary adventure.

5. Inflammation is reduced. The persistent immune response brought on by celiac disease means chronic inflammation in the body. Going gluten-free means that immune reaction is halted and inflammation is reduced.

Gluten-Free Kids

Giving up favorite foods is difficult for everyone, but especially for children too young to understand the health hazard that gluten poses. My best tip is to demonstrate to kids (and others) that gluten-free food can taste even better than traditional recipes. That's where the recipes I created for you will save the day. Get the kids in the kitchen and whip up a pizza in 30 minutes. Bake brownies for the school bake sale. Make a loaf of bread for sandwiches. Don't be discouraged if your child doesn't love everything you make. Kids can be picky . . . and brutally honest.

Highlight for kids the naturally gluten-free foods they already love. Stock up on healthier gluten-free snacks like popcorn and fruit snacks. Volunteer to bake the class party cupcakes. Tuck a gluten-free snack in your purse or car so you always have something ready to eat for your young one. The more gluten-free–friendly you keep your life, the easier the adjustments will be.

Gluten Intolerance on the Rise

Humans have been eating wheat and enjoying the gluten it contains for 10,000 years. Before we had a reason to avoid it, most of us never gave gluten a second thought. Now that it demands our attention, let's take a look at some facts.

Since 1950, the incidence of celiac disease has quadrupled. This could be due to:

- Increased awareness in the medical community
- Heightened public awareness of the disease
- Improved testing measures for celiac disease

Although some people suggest that the wheat we eat today is vastly different from the wheat grown 100 years ago, research does not support this idea. There isn't a significant difference in the actual wheat plant or in its gluten content.

What has changed is this:

- The wheat products we eat are more processed now, resulting in more gluten and fewer nutrients (as in white wheat flour).
- Our diets include more refined, processed foods, many of which contain gluten. This change has occurred far faster than our bodies can adapt.
- The gut microbiome (the bacteria that keeps us healthy) has changed over time.

With all these factors, is it any wonder so many of us have a gluten intolerance?

Gluten, Gluten Everywhere

Living a gluten-free life involves more than avoiding bread. Often we overlook foods with "hidden" gluten or cross-contamination, not to mention cookware and utensils that might harbor gluten. Knowing where to look and what to look for goes a long way in managing a gluten-free lifestyle.

GLUTEN IN FOOD AND FOOD PRODUCTS

Gluten shows up in more foods than wheat. Other grains like barley and rye contain gluten. Unless they are specified as purity protocol grown, oats are also off-limits. Sometimes, wheat and other gluten-containing grains go by other names, further confusing matters. Even food additives like flavors and colors can be a source of gluten.

In other cases, gluten is not directly added, but enters by way of cross-contamination. That is when an otherwise gluten-free food is exposed to gluten. Cross-contamination can occur anywhere. For example:

- In food manufacturing, when gluten-free and gluten-containing products are produced in the same facility and when shared equipment is used to produce or package foods.

- In the home kitchen, when we use shared cutting boards, utensils, and even hand towels or dish sponges. Condiments and spreads (peanut butter, jam, etc.) are often assumed to be gluten-free, but when a utensil used for one of these foods touches regular bread and ends up back in the jar, the entire jar is contaminated. Toasters and cookware obviously do not naturally contain gluten, but can become contaminated with it. If you toast gluten-free bread in a toaster used for regular bread, there's a good chance lingering gluten-filled crumbs will end up on your bread and in your body. Chapter two goes into more detail about how to set up your kitchen to be a safe gluten-free space.

- In grocery stores, when deli slicers are shared, in bulk bin foods, and at salad bars where spills occur and serving utensils are shared. Another potentially risky item is a repackaged food, such as cheese that is cut from a large wheel, then rewrapped for sale. If this is done in the part of the store where gluten products are used, there could be cross-contamination.

Letting Gluten Go

The feelings associated with giving up gluten are sometimes compared with the five stages of grief. Those stages are:

- Denial
- Anger
- Bargaining
- Depression
- Acceptance

Few of us want to accept a flaw in the system that prevents us from eating common, familiar foods. The forced change of having to give up gluten, and seeing others continue to enjoy those foods we can no longer have, can be frustrating. However, in time, most of us realize a gluten-free diet is not so restrictive. It becomes easier to manage over time, and the health benefits are worth it.

Everyone is unique, and so is the experience of going gluten-free. Honor your feelings, both negative and positive. I experienced my share of emotions after my celiac diagnosis. Mostly, I felt relief. After 25 years of chronic pain and dozens of misdiagnoses, having a name for it (celiac disease) and a solution (gluten-free diet) meant I could restore my health. No more mystery illnesses, no more doctors telling me it was all in my head, and no more feeling sick all the time.

When grocery shopping, look for the words *gluten-free* on the package. But, because even that is not always a guarantee, read every ingredient. Foods that contain wheat (or any other of the top eight allergens) will disclose it in a statement below the ingredients list. If you aren't sure about an ingredient and an online search doesn't answer the question, you should contact the manufacturer.

Use the following lists to guide your food choices and steer clear of gluten. Please know that *these lists are not all-inclusive*, but provide an overview of which regular foods and drinks commonly include gluten.

Any food containing wheat, barley, rye, or regular oats contains gluten. Some may seem obvious; others may not. My focus is on mainstream foods, not specialty versions made to be gluten-free.

- Beer, hard cider, wine coolers
- Black licorice
- Breaded or battered foods
- Bread crumbs, panko (Japanese bread crumbs)
- Breads like bagels, muffins, rolls, pita, naan, flatbread, cornbread (or dry mixes)
- Brewer's yeast
- Cakes, cookies, brownies, donuts (or dry mixes)
- Canned soup
- Cereal, granola, granola bars
- Crackers, pretzels
- Croutons
- Dry sauce mixes
- Dumplings
- Fish-fry batter mix
- Gravy (prepared and dry mix)
- Imitation crab, seafood, bacon bits
- Miso
- Noodles (ramen, udon, etc.)
- Pie crust, puff pastry
- Protein bars
- Red "licorice" candy (such as Twizzlers or Red Vines)
- Soy sauce
- Tabbouleh
- Tempura
- Tortillas (flour)

FOODS THAT MIGHT HAVE GLUTEN—CHECK LABELS

Not every food listed here contains gluten and, for most, it is relatively easy to find a gluten-free version; however, sometimes foods we expect to be gluten-free surprise us. For example, some highly processed cold cuts contain wheat starch as a binder. Pay careful attention to the following foods, which might contain gluten:

- Canned soups
- Cheese (typically gluten-free, but varieties with added seasonings, herbs, spices, and some blue cheeses could contain gluten)
- Chewing gum (sometimes has wheat starch used as a binder)
- Cold cuts (highly processed cold cuts could use gluten as a binder)

- Corn products (cornstarch, cornmeal, grits, polenta, etc. may contain gluten via cross-contact with gluten grains in the field and/or during processing)
- Dry herbs and spice blends (sometimes use wheat starch as an anticaking agent)
- Frozen vegetables with added sauce or seasoning
- Marinades, bottled
- Meats and poultry, pre-marinated
- Oats, unless specified "grown with gluten-free purity protocol"
- Potato chips (varieties with seasonings may contain wheat starch or malt for flavoring)
- Salad dressings (may use wheat starch as a binder; malt is sometimes used as flavoring)
- Soy flour

Start Simply

Now that you've bid gluten farewell and learned where it might be lurking, think about the delicious possibilities that await. You may miss gluten for a while—I sure did—but in time your health will improve, and you'll be excited about how easy it is to create delicious gluten-free meals at home. When I started living gluten-free, a simple approach worked best. It helped me adapt to my new way of eating. I learned a few tricks along the way that made gluten-free cooking (and eating!) something I now look forward to every day.

Eat naturally gluten-free food. Lean meats, poultry and fish, fresh fruit and vegetables, nuts and seeds, dairy products, and eggs are naturally gluten-free. They can be part of an overall nutritious diet with no added expense, since they are not specialty items.

Use recipes with few ingredients and short cooking times. One of my main goals in writing this book was to develop recipes with short ingredient lists and/or short prep and cook times. As a busy working mom, I relate to that "too tired to cook" feeling at day's end. That's why I'm happy to show you it's possible to get meals on the table fast. It's even possible to make pancakes for breakfast and dessert on weeknights without feeling rushed.

Meal prep. I spend about four hours one day each week in my kitchen prepping a full week's worth of foods—breakfasts, lunches, and dinners. Many of the recipes I'm sharing here are ones I prep ahead. When it's time to make dinner, I'm not at a loss for what to make. It's easy to pull together roasted veggies and leftovers from a roast and then whip up a naturally gluten-free dessert in no time. It takes the guesswork out of the meals for the week and the stress out of meal planning.

Gluten by Many Other Names

Derivatives of wheat, barley, rye, and regular oats must be avoided on a gluten-free diet, too. Because "gluten" is not listed as an ingredient on food labels, nor is it called out in an allergen statement (only wheat is), it is helpful to be familiar with the various names of gluten-containing grains and grain-based products. They include:

- Atta
- Bulgur
- Dinkle
- Durum
- Einkorn
- Emmer
- Farina
- Farro (Faro)
- Fu
- Graham
- Kamut
- Maltose
- Malt syrup, extract, flavoring
- Malt vinegar
- Pumpernickel
- Seitan
- Semolina
- Spelt
- Triga
- Triticale

Focus on Healthy

Healthy means something different to everyone. For me, healthy living encompasses every aspect of life—mind, body, and spirit. Food plays a significant role in each of those. Fueling up on foods we love that provide energy for our bodies is essential.

I found that, to heal my digestive system and improve overall health, eating mostly naturally gluten-free foods like fresh vegetables, fruits, and lean proteins is best. I minimize highly processed gluten-free foods and avoid buying products with long ingredient lists, which usually indicate many chemical additives. Although it may be exciting to see a gluten-free version of your favorite packaged food, just remember that gluten-free doesn't necessarily equal healthy. Gluten-free packaged products are as likely to be laden with sugar, highly refined fats, excess sodium, and additives as their traditional counterparts.

Here are my top five tips for healthy gluten-free eating:

1. Follow the 90–10 rule. Make 90 percent of what you eat naturally gluten-free. Reserve treats made with alternative flours for special occasions.

2. Meet daily fruit and vegetable requirements. Getting enough plants into your diet is essential for optimal health.

3. Limit packaged foods. Most gluten-free packaged foods contain xanthan gum and other additives that can cause digestive issues.

4. Balance daily food intake. If you enjoy toast at breakfast and a sandwich at lunch, skip the rolls at dinner. Keep a balance of protein, healthy fats, and carbohydrates for sustained energy.

5. Eat in-season foods as much as possible. This adds variety to your diet and ensures that you consume a variety of nutrients.

Approach Baking Patiently

When you're new to gluten-free living, gluten-free baking is uncharted territory. Even accomplished bakers are stymied by the new, often esoteric rules of gluten-free baking. Be patient with yourself as you learn how to work with novel ingredients. Traditional notions about baking are out the window. Most batters will look different. Instead of kneading bread, your mixer will stir the batter for you, then it will go right into the pan. Cake batter will seem too thin. Cookie dough may appear too thick. Don't let these differences hold you back. It might take some trial and error to get baked goods right, but the following tips and techniques will help.

Test your oven temperature. Oven temperatures vary. Purchase an inexpensive oven thermometer and hang it in the center of your oven. Set the oven temperature to 350°F and wait 20 minutes to read the thermometer. Adjust your oven's temperature if needed by following the manufacturer's directions.

Use the correct pan. Pan size and material matter. A pan that is too large leads to overcooked foods. One that's too small leaves foods undercooked. When baking sweets, like brownies, use a metal pan. Recipes with a high sugar content brown too quickly in a glass dish.

Addressing Other Allergens

Living gluten-free can seem overwhelming at first, but being faced with additional food allergies or intolerances makes meals even more complicated. Because I understand personally what it is like to live with celiac disease and multiple food allergies, I created the recipes in this book to be as allergen-friendly as possible. In addition to being gluten-free, every recipe is free from soy, peanuts, and tree nuts. Coconut is used in many of the recipes, but it is not a tree nut, despite being labeled as such by the FDA.

All but fifteen recipes are dairy-free, and 100 recipes are egg-free. Most recipes have at least one variation, as well as substitution options for allergens when possible, making this collection one of the most versatile available.

Measure flour properly. See the discussion of scales on page 23. To measure flour by volume, spoon it into a measuring cup, allowing it to heap up, then use a flat edge to sweep across the top of the measuring cup to level.

Follow the recipe as written. In recipes for soups or casseroles, tweaks here and there are fine. But baking is a precise process. First, make the recipe as written to see the intended results; then you have a baseline from which to adjust.

Follow directions all the way through. This includes cooling time after baking. Foods continue to cook once they're removed from the oven, and some recipes allow for this with shorter baking times and a prescribed cooling period in the pan.

Change one ingredient at a time. If you modify a recipe, make one ingredient change at a time. This helps you know how that change affected the outcome. Changing more than one ingredient prevents you from knowing which change made the difference.

If a recipe doesn't go as planned, here are some ideas for using your not-quite-perfect results:

- Cake tastes great but sinks in the center or crumbles apart? Cut it into cubes and make a trifle (layers of cake, pudding, whipped cream, and fruit).

- Cookies spread into one huge cookie on the pan? Cool, crumble, and store them in a sealed container to use as a crumble on your next ice cream dessert.

- Bread tastes fine but the texture is not quite right? Cut it into cubes, toast in the oven, cool, and put it in your food processor to make bread crumbs.

My best advice to you is to approach your gluten-free baking with confidence, trust the recipes as written, and keep your sense of humor.

This Book's Recipes

When deciding which recipes to include, I thought back to those early days after my celiac disease diagnosis. My approach to home cooking has always been about being practical, efficient, and time-conscious. It's important to me to eat well without breaking the bank. That didn't change after my diagnosis.

At the beginning of each chapter, I share the essential information you need to make the recipes in that chapter. Throughout the book, you will find a mix of naturally gluten-free dishes, transformed old favorites, and plenty of recipes for holidays and special occasions.

Chapter 3 contains essential recipes like Pizza Crust (page 29) and Flour Tortillas (page 36) that can be used on their own and in other recipes. The remaining chapters are divided by type of dish, with two dessert chapters. In chapter 13, Cookies, Cakes & More, you'll find recipes for beloved baked goods like carrot cake, brownies, and cupcakes that I transformed into gluten-free versions you won't believe taste as good as they do. In chapter 14, Naturally Gluten-Free Desserts, the recipes are more fruit-forward, like Inside-Out Caramel Baked Apples (page 229) and Poached Pears with Butterscotch Sauce (page 226). I also didn't forget my fellow chocolate lovers! My irresistible Vegan Double-Chocolate Pudding (page 228) recipe just happens to be naturally gluten-free.

As mentioned before, *all the recipes are free from gluten, soy, peanuts, and tree nuts.* Recipes that are dairy-free or egg-free—or have substitution options in the ingredient lists that would make them so—are noted as such at the beginning of the recipe.
In fact, only 15 of the 160 recipes in this book require dairy for the best results. The remaining 145 recipes are either already dairy-free or have a simple substitute. There are 100 egg-free recipes in this book, too. If a recipe is vegan or vegetarian, that's noted as well. Recipe labels also include 5 Ingredients or Less (not including cooking oil or butter, water, salt, and black pepper), 30 Minutes or Less (from start to finish), No Cook (recipes that require no cooking at all), and One Pot (indicating the use of just one pot or dish or bowl), so that you can easily select recipes that suit busy weeknights.

To keep it interesting, most recipes include a variation or two that change up flavors or provide an alternative for other allergens. You'll also find a wealth of tips for finding ingredients, making substitutions, and prepping ahead. And I include product recommendations when I have a preference for a particular brand.

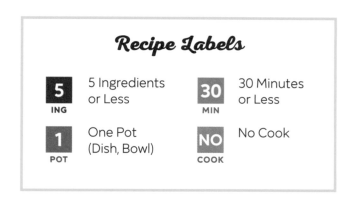

Recipe Labels

5 ING — 5 Ingredients or Less

30 MIN — 30 Minutes or Less

1 POT — One Pot (Dish, Bowl)

NO COOK — No Cook

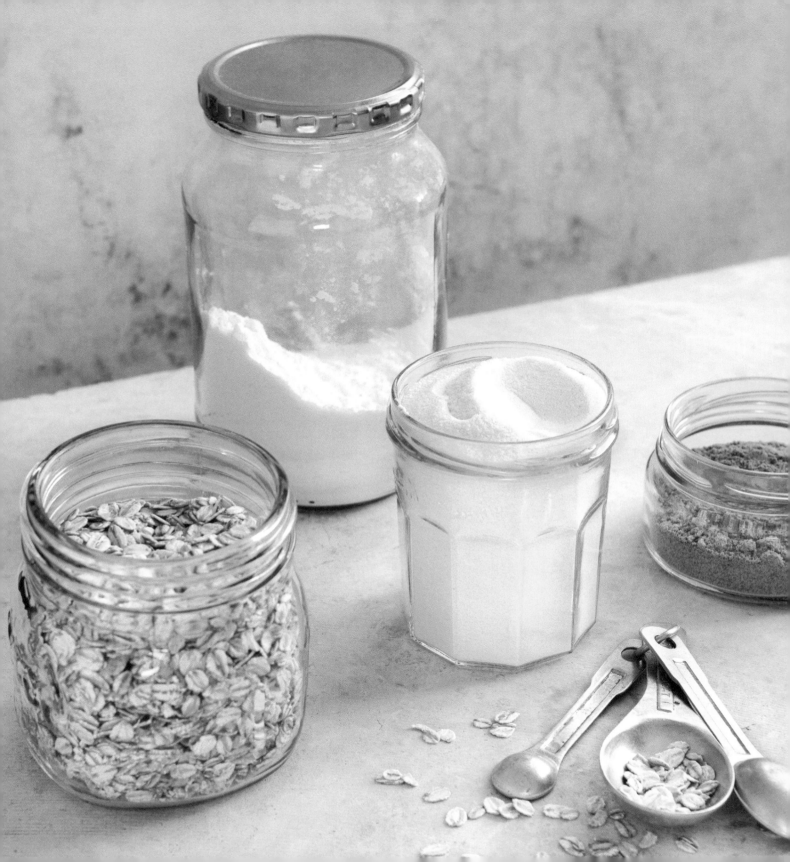

CHAPTER 2

Your Gluten-Free Kitchen

There's more to a gluten-free lifestyle than changing our diet. For those of us with celiac disease or another gluten-related health issue, we are on constant alert for gluten. Every aspect of life is affected by our need to avoid gluten, including kitchen organization. If you live alone, setting up and maintaining a fully gluten-free kitchen is an easy decision. But if there are others in the house to consider, that usually means compromise. After all, try telling your kids their favorite cookies are suddenly off-limits. The tips and strategies in this chapter will help you figure out what works best in your home.

After my celiac diagnosis in 2007, my husband suggested we keep an entirely gluten-free kitchen. Having watched me suffer for years with poor health, he was eager to help me heal. Our children were young enough that they didn't realize the changes. My previous work in recipe development made re-creating favorite recipes less daunting. However, everyone's situation differs. A completely gluten-free kitchen isn't always possible. If that's the case for you, don't worry. With the right precautions, a shared kitchen can work.

The Shared Kitchen

Cross-contamination is the primary issue with shared space. Separate storage areas are needed for the refrigerator, freezer, and pantry. Consider designated shelves for gluten-free foods (above gluten-containing foods in case of spills). Even a small morsel of gluten contamination is problematic, especially for anyone with celiac disease. Small plastic bins are a good option to segregate foods.

Cutting boards, colanders, porous utensils (like wooden spoons), some cookware (like cast iron and clay), and plastic storage containers can all harbor gluten. Toasters, waffle irons, and griddles can hold onto crumbs. Dish sponges and hand towels can, too. Invest in new items and dedicate them for exclusive use with gluten-free foods. Color coding (green for gluten-free, red for gluten, for example) helps keep items separate.

Beyond food prep and cooking items, consider anything gluten could touch, such as countertops, tables, doorknobs, and faucets. If someone eats a regular sandwich and touches those surfaces, they become potential gluten hot spots. Washing these surfaces after every use minimizes cross-contamination.

It's a big investment in time and money, but keep in mind, you only need to set up your kitchen once . . . and this is for your health. Help everyone in your home understand this, review the new kitchen procedures (post them on the refrigerator if you need to), and be diligent in the process.

Pantry Essentials

After your kitchen is organized, it's time for the fun part—stocking your pantry! Imagine how easy it will be to make your favorite meals with all the essentials at your fingertips. Stocking your most-used ingredients prevents last-minute trips to the grocery store for a forgotten item, helps you get a nourishing meal on the table faster, and even makes your regular grocery shopping easier. Your initial pantry stocking list is likely to be a long one, but once that's done, your weekly grocery list will consist of main ingredients like meats and fresh produce. What's even better? Knowing which items you use regularly means you can stock up when those items are on sale.

A well-stocked pantry is a useful approach for any home cook and is especially important for those of us on a gluten-free diet. Before going gluten-free, if there was nothing to make for dinner at the end of a long day, my husband and I would go to a

Flours, Meals, and Starches

Ingredient names can be confusing. Let's tackle a few that are used in this book.

Cornmeal versus Cornstarch: Cornmeal is dried corn with the germ and bran removed. Most recipes for cornbread use finely ground cornmeal. Cornstarch (corn flour) is the starch extracted from corn. It is used to thicken soups, stews, puddings, and gravies.

Flaxseeds, Flaxseed Meal, and Chia Seeds: Flaxseeds are whole seeds; flaxseed meal is ground seeds. Chia seeds are always whole. One tablespoon of flax meal or chia seeds stirred into 3 tablespoons warm water equals one large egg. You can use this as a substitute for up to 2 large eggs in recipes like cookies and muffins for egg-free baking.

Potato Starch versus Potato Flour: Potato starch is used in my flour blend (page 27). It has a neutral flavor and lightens the texture of baked goods. It also thickens gravies and sauces. You can substitute potato starch for cornstarch in an equal quantity as a thickener. Potato flour is made from whole potatoes (versus only the starch) and has a distinct potato flavor. It readily absorbs liquid and can lead to dry or gummy baked goods. No recipes in this book use potato flour.

favorite restaurant or order takeout without a second thought. On a gluten-free diet, simply finding a restaurant where you feel safe eating can take longer than it would to prepare a meal if your pantry contained all the essentials.

I created the recipes in this book with a well-stocked gluten-free pantry in mind, avoiding single-use ingredients or items that aren't budget-friendly. After all, I'm a busy mom with celiac disease and multiple food allergies.

The following list is a peek inside my pantry. It contains the essential ingredients to create the recipes in this book, as well as items that will help you create the variations I provide. Of course, every item is gluten-free. I include dairy-free ingredients in the list as well, but if you don't have a problem with dairy, you can choose whether to include them in your pantry. I always buy organic when available, but do what works for you. To make stocking your pantry as easy as possible, I've compiled a list of my favorite brands, which you can find on page 239.

Always check every label on the items you buy to make sure they are gluten-free and free from any allergens you must avoid. Manufacturers can (and do) change ingredients, sourcing, and recipes, so even if you buy an item regularly, always double-check the label.

FLOURS AND STARCHES

- Arrowroot starch (also called arrowroot flour, arrowroot powder)
- Guar gum
- Potato starch
- Rice flour: brown or white
- Tapioca flour (also called tapioca starch)

GRAINS, PASTA, AND BEANS

- Beans and peas: canned and/or dried (black, black-eyed peas, chickpeas)
- Cornmeal, finely ground
- Gluten-free pasta: manicotti, spaghetti, elbows, and penne
- Oats, rolled, grown with a gluten-free purity protocol
- Quinoa
- Rice: brown, white, wild

OILS AND OTHER FATS

- Butter, ghee, or dairy-free butter
- Palm shortening
- Oils: avocado oil or coconut oil (for high-heat sautéing and for greasing pans); sunflower oil (for baking)

CANS, BOTTLES, JARS, BOXES

- Applesauce, unsweetened
- Coconut aminos (or gluten-free soy sauce)
- Coconut milk: boxed unsweetened, canned full-fat, canned light (or other plant- or dairy-based milk of your choice)
- Hot sauce
- Mustard: prepared yellow and Dijon
- Pineapple, crushed, in its own juice
- Pumpkin purée
- Stock: vegetable, chicken, and beef
- Nut or seed butter
- Tahini (sesame seed paste)
- Tomatoes: diced, crushed, and whole
- Tomato paste
- Vinegar: balsamic, apple cider, and rice

SPICES AND SEASONINGS

- Black pepper
- Cayenne pepper, ground
- Chili powder
- Chives, dried
- Cilantro, dried
- Cinnamon, ground
- Cumin, ground
- Dill, dried (also called dill weed)
- Garlic powder (not garlic salt)
- Onion powder (not onion salt)
- Sage, ground (also called rubbed sage)
- Salt: regular table salt (for baking) and coarse sea salt (for finishing dishes)
- Turmeric, ground

ADDITIONAL BAKING INGREDIENTS

- Baking powder, aluminum-free
- Baking soda
- Chocolate: dark or semisweet; chips or chunks
- Cocoa powder, unsweetened
- Coconut, dried, unsweetened
- Coconut milk powder
- Dates: Medjool (for cooking); Deglet Noor (for snacking)
- Honey
- Maple syrup, pure
- Nuts and/or seeds
- Sugar: granulated, light brown, coconut sugar, and confectioners (powdered)
- Vanilla extract, pure
- Yeast, fast-acting

A Note on Gums

Gluten provides elasticity and texture in baked goods. Removing gluten means adding something—usually gum—to mimic those qualities. But because they can be irritating to the digestive system, I avoid using gums whenever possible. Fortunately, most recipes in the book do not require the addition of gum; however, gum is necessary in yeast breads, so I use a small amount of guar gum. Guar is plant-derived, whereas xanthan gum is harvested from lab-grown, bacteria-fed sugar derived from corn, wheat, or soy. Although xanthan gum is considered gluten-free and allergen-free, it is difficult to determine the source of the feeding sugar, which is a concern for individuals with food allergies.

If you use a flour blend instead of either the gum-free blend in this book (Gigi's Everyday Gluten-Free Flour, page 27) or the recommended store-bought gum-free equivalent, make sure your choice does not contain gum. My recipes are designed with ingredients that work together, so the addition of gum is not required. If a blend with gum is used in a recipe that does not call for gum, your baked goods will be gummy, seem undercooked, and/or may sink in the center.

Kitchen Favorites

I stock my refrigerator and pantry with items that complement one another. If you do, too, you'll get into your own food groove, flex with the seasons, and find that meals come together very quickly. In spring and summer, my meals are more plant-centered and I use fewer pantry items. In fall and winter, I buy more organic canned pumpkin, coconut milk, and canned tomatoes, because those ingredients work best with what's in season near me. Peek inside my refrigerator and freezer and here's what you'll find:

FROZEN FOODS

- Berries (blackberries, blueberries, strawberries, etc.)
- Broccoli
- Brussels sprouts
- Cauliflower: florets and riced
- Collard greens
- Corn
- Green peas
- Mushrooms

REFRIGERATED FOODS

- Bacon, uncured, natural
- Broccoli
- Butter, dairy-free
- Cabbage
- Carrots
- Cauliflower
- Cheese: goat, Cheddar, Gouda, Parmesan, mozzarella, for dairy lovers (and dairy-free for me)
- Cilantro
- Cucumbers, Persian
- Eggs, organic, pasture-raised
- Hummus
- Jalapeño peppers, pickled
- Jam (apricot, strawberry) and marmalade
- Mayonnaise
- Milk, unsweetened coconut
- Mushrooms
- Olives: green, black, and Kalamata
- Salad greens
- Smoked salmon
- Sour cream, full-fat
- Spinach
- Strawberries (in season only)
- Yogurt, plain: plant-based and dairy-based
- Zucchini

OTHER FOODS

There's also a handful of produce I regularly use that does not need refrigeration or freezer storage, including:

- Apples
- Avocados
- Bananas
- Garlic
- Gingerroot
- Lemons
- Limes
- Pears
- Potatoes: white and sweet
- Tomatoes
- Turnips

STORING FRESH HERBS

Fresh herbs add so much flavor to meals, but many of us use just a portion and end up discarding the rest once it's gone bad. Here are some tips for extending the life of these foods.

- For fresh herbs like basil, cilantro, and parsley, wash them in cool water, lightly shake off excess water, then spread out on paper towels. Pat with additional paper towels and air dry, uncovered. Once completely dry, roll them up in a clean paper towel and place in a large zip-top bag. Squeeze out the air from the bag, label, and refrigerate in the vegetable bin. Herbs will last up to two weeks.

- For prewashed salad greens, layer them on paper towels, roll up loosely, and store in a large zip-top bag. Squeeze out the air from the bag, label, and refrigerate in the vegetable bin for up to one week.

- For fresh ginger, peel, slice, and store it in the freezer in freezer-safe containers or plastic bags for up to three months. Thaw at room temperature when ready to use.

Kitchen Equipment

To successfully create the recipes in this book, there are certain pieces of kitchen equipment you must have and other items that are nice to have:

MUST-HAVES

- Baking sheets (2)
- Blender
- Cutting boards (2)
- Digital kitchen scale
- Digital thermometer
- Loaf pan
- Muffin tin

NICE-TO-HAVES

- Food processor
- Immersion (stick) blender
- Mini muffin tin
- Slow cooker, pressure cooker, or multicooker (slow cooker/pressure cooker combo)
- Spiral slicer

Don't Fear the Scale

Digital scales are inexpensive and make baking easier by yielding consistently accurate results. I use metric measurements when I bake. To weigh ingredients for baking, set the scale measurement to grams. Place a bowl on the scale and tare the scale before adding the ingredient. Taring sets the scale to zero so the weight of the bowl is not counted in the measurement. Add the ingredient to the bowl and note the weight.

You can measure all dry ingredients for a recipe in a single bowl. To do this, tare the scale after each ingredient and repeat until all dry ingredients are weighed.

If you prefer to measure by volume, gently spoon the dry ingredient into a measuring cup, allowing it to heap up. Use the back edge of a butter knife to level the flour at the top of the measuring cup. Do not plunge a measuring cup into dry ingredients to scoop them. This packs them into the measuring cup and will throw off your measurement, usually resulting in dry baked goods.

CHAPTER 3

Essentials

Every great home cook has a collection of recipes they consider essentials. These are recipes you turn to repeatedly because they work well on their own, but also because they are foundation recipes for other dishes. The essential recipes in this chapter are designed to set up anyone—new or seasoned cook—for success in the kitchen. With these basics in your repertoire, you're halfway home to a delicious meal.

Recipes like these are the cornerstones of many recipes throughout the book, and they are versatile enough to use in your own favorite dishes. From a reliable gluten-free flour blend and quick baking mix, to sauces, seasonings, and homemade stock, these recipes can inspire many meals and help you get dinner on the table quickly.

Prep time: 10 minutes

NO COOK · 30 MIN

960 grams (about 6 cups)
Gigi's Everyday Gluten-
Free Flour (page 27)

50 grams (about ¼ cup)
baking powder

27 grams (about
2 tablespoons) sugar

18 grams (about
1 tablespoon) salt

6 grams (about
½ tablespoon) guar gum

Quick Baking Mix

Vegan Use this mix as you would a store-bought quick baking mix. The perks of making this mix yourself are that it's super easy to whisk together, saves you lots of money, and is free from the additives and excess sodium you find in commercial mixes. It's also a great time-saver when making recipes like pancakes and waffles.

1. In a large bowl, whisk together all the ingredients until well blended.

2. Store in an airtight glass container in the pantry for up to 3 months, or in the refrigerator for up to 6 months.

PER SERVING (¼ cup): Calories: 130; Total fat: 1g; Total carbs: 31g; Sugar: 1g; Protein: 2g; Fiber: 1g; Sodium: 272mg

Prep time: 10 minutes

325 grams (about
2½ cups) brown
rice flour

113 grams (about 1 cup)
tapioca starch

150 grams (about 1 cup)
potato starch
(not potato flour)

32 grams (about ¼ cup)
arrowroot starch

Gigi's Everyday Gluten-Free Flour

Vegan This versatile flour blend is a budget-saver. It's far less expensive than store-bought blends. Although gums are common in gluten-free recipes, they aren't always necessary. Where gums are required for optimal results, the recipe will call for them. If you do not bake often or prefer a premade blend, King Arthur Gluten-Free All-Purpose Flour—without added gum—is an exact swap for this one.

1. Combine all the ingredients in a large bowl; whisk to blend thoroughly.

2. Store in an airtight glass container at room temperature for up to 3 months. Alternatively, refrigerate for up to 6 months.

MAKE-AHEAD TIP *If you bake often, double the recipe to make 9½ cups.*

SUBSTITUTION TIP *Brown rice flour is slightly more nutritious and flavorful than white rice flour, but the two are interchangeable in their baking properties.*

PER SERVING (35 grams, about ¼ cup): Calories: 135; Total fat: 1g; Total carbs: 31g; Sugar: 0g; Protein: 2g; Fiber: 1g; Sodium: 2mg

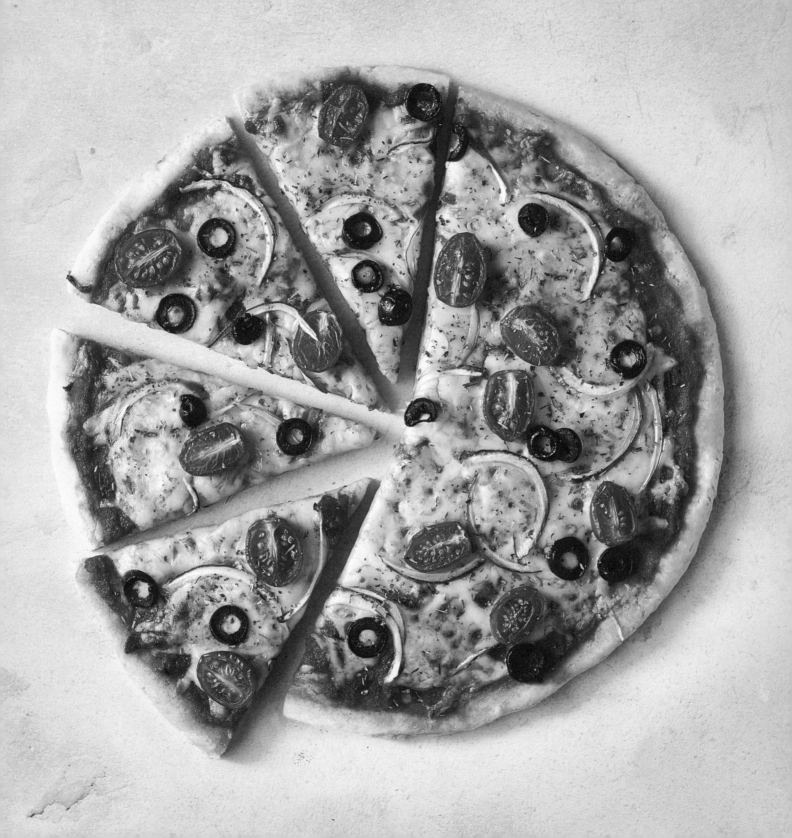

MAKES 1 (12-INCH) PIZZA CRUST

Prep time: 10 minutes plus 15 minutes to rise

Cook time: 20 minutes

300 grams (about 2 cups) Gigi's Everyday Gluten-Free Flour (page 27)

½ teaspoon salt

2 teaspoons guar gum

2 tablespoons neutral oil, such as sunflower, plus additional to grease your hands

1 cup warm (108° to 110°F) water

10 grams (about 2½ teaspoons) fast-acting yeast

1 teaspoon granulated sugar

Pizza Crust

Vegan If you miss a tender pizza crust, with just the right amount of snap and real yeasty flavor, fire up the oven! You can mix this dough by hand, shape the crust on the pan, and bake it after a quick 15-minute rise. Adjust the size of the dough according to your preference for thicker or thinner crust, or divide the dough and shape it into individual pizzas.

TO MAKE THE DOUGH

1. If making the dough to use right away, preheat the oven to 450°F and line a round pizza pan with parchment paper. If making the dough in advance to freeze, skip this step and see the make-ahead tip.

2. In a medium bowl, whisk together the flour and salt.

3. In a small bowl, whisk together the guar gum and oil until smooth.

4. In a measuring cup or separate small bowl, combine the warm water, yeast, and sugar. Set aside and allow the yeast to proof (ferment), undisturbed, for 5 minutes.

5. Once the yeast mixture appears frothy on top, pour it into the flour, then add the guar gum-oil mixture. Stir until well combined and a dough forms. If saving it for later, wrap the dough tightly in plastic wrap and refrigerate overnight. When ready to use, proceed with the next steps.

➤

TO BAKE THE DOUGH

1. Preheat the oven if you have not yet done it. Rub a small amount of the oil between your hands. Place the dough on the pizza pan and shape into a large circle, about 12 inches in diameter, forming a slight edge around the pizza, if you like.

2. Place a piece of wax paper lightly over the top of the dough (do not press down) and let the crust rise for 15 minutes. Discard the wax paper.

3. Place the crust in the oven and bake for 10 minutes. Remove the crust from the oven, add sauce, cheese, and other desired toppings, then return your pizza to the oven for 10 minutes more.

VARIATION **Garlic Parmesan Crust:** Add 3 minced garlic cloves and ½ cup of grated Parmesan cheese to the dough along with the ingredients in step 5. Proceed as directed.

MAKE-AHEAD TIP *To freeze the dough, add 5 grams (about 1 teaspoon) of additional yeast in step 4 and prepare through step 5. Cover the dough completely on top with greased plastic wrap. (Freeze the dough on the pan to maintain its shape.) Once frozen solid, remove it from the pan and completely wrap it again in plastic wrap to keep it fresh. Freeze for up to 1 month. Thaw at room temperature, uncover, and bake as directed in step 3.*

PER SERVING (⅛ crust): Calories: 175; Total fat: 3g; Total carbs: 32g; Sugar: 0g; Protein: 3g; Fiber: 2g; Sodium: 146mg

Five-Minute Pizza/Pasta Sauce

MAKES ABOUT 2 CUPS

Prep time: 10 minutes

COOK · MIN

1 (15-ounce) can diced tomatoes, drained

1 medium carrot, cut into 2-inch pieces (1 cup), or 10 baby carrots

¼ cup fresh basil leaves

1 garlic clove, minced

1 teaspoon balsamic vinegar

1 teaspoon sugar (optional)

1 teaspoon dried oregano

¼ teaspoon salt

5 grinds freshly ground black pepper

Dairy-free · Egg-free · Vegan When my daughters were growing up, we couldn't find a pizza sauce they both liked. Even the best restaurant pizzas failed their "picky palate" test. I did the only thing I could do—created a healthy pizza sauce the entire family loved. This fresh, fast, and flavorful sauce is still our go-to recipe. It works well on pasta, too.

1. Combine all the ingredients in a blender or food processor and blend until smooth.

2. Use as a pizza sauce or warm it and toss with cooked pasta or zucchini noodles.

VARIATION 1 Classic Italian Pasta Sauce: Use red wine vinegar in place of the balsamic and add 3 tablespoons extra-virgin olive oil and a pinch of red pepper flakes.

VARIATION 2 Creamy Red Sauce: Omit the basil leaves and sugar and add ¼ cup heavy (whipping) cream or canned coconut milk (for dairy-free) and 1 tablespoon of butter (or ghee or dairy-free butter).

ALLERGEN TIP *If you cannot eat carrots, use 2 cups chopped cooked beets instead for a rich, brilliantly colored sauce.*

PER SERVING (¼ cup): Calories: 17; Total fat: 0g; Total carbs: 4g; Sugar: 2g; Protein: 1g; Fiber: 1g; Sodium: 154mg

Prep time: 5 minutes

Cook time: 10 minutes

1½ cups chicken stock
or water

10 Medjool dates, pitted

1 (6-ounce) can
tomato paste

¼ cup gluten-free
soy sauce

4 tablespoons
yellow mustard

3 tablespoons
rice vinegar

Juice of ½ lemon

1 tablespoon ghee

2 teaspoons
garlic powder

2 teaspoons
onion powder

2 teaspoons hot sauce

1 teaspoon
dried oregano

1 teaspoon chopped
chipotle in adobo sauce

½ teaspoon salt

¼ teaspoon chili powder

All-American Barbecue Sauce

Egg-free Commercial barbecue sauces tend to be high in sugar, since sweetness is needed to balance flavors from ingredients like vinegar and spicy peppers. In place of sugar, I use high-fiber, nutrient-dense dates, which are a low glycemic food. The sauce still has a sweet balance without sending your blood sugar soaring. Use this sauce anywhere you normally use barbecue sauce. Try it on the Barbecue Chicken Pizza (page 169).

1. Combine all the ingredients in a blender and blend until smooth, then transfer the sauce to a medium saucepan. Alternatively, place the ingredients in a medium saucepan and use an immersion blender to blend until smooth.

2. Place the saucepan over medium-high heat and cook just until the sauce is about to boil. Reduce the heat to low, cover, and simmer for 10 minutes.

3. Remove from heat and let the sauce cool completely to allow the flavors to come together.

4. Store in an airtight glass container for up to 2 weeks in the refrigerator, or up to 1 month in the freezer.

VARIATION **South Carolina–Style Mustard Sauce:** Omit the tomato paste, soy sauce, lemon juice, oregano, and chili powder. Reduce the stock to ½ cup and increase the mustard to ¾ cup. Instead of rice vinegar, use ¼ cup apple cider vinegar.

SUBSTITUTION TIP *Replace the stock with water and the ghee with vegan butter to make this recipe vegan. If you are allergic to soy, substitute coconut aminos for the soy sauce.*

PER SERVING (2 tablespoons): Calories: 65; Total fat: 1g; Total carbs: 15g; Sugar: 11g; Protein: 1g; Fiber: 2g; Sodium: 92mg

**MAKES ABOUT
1¾ CUPS**

Prep time: 5 minutes

NO COOK | 30 MIN

1 cup coconut
milk powder

2 tablespoons
dried cilantro

2 tablespoons
garlic powder

2 tablespoons
onion powder

2 tablespoons
dried chives

1 tablespoon dried dill

2 teaspoons salt

½ teaspoon freshly
ground white pepper

Homemade Ranch Seasoning

Vegan Use this mix for salad dressings, dips, seasonings, and more. Coconut milk powder is a versatile and inexpensive ingredient that works well for those of us who must be dairy-free. Be sure to run it through a sieve to remove clumps before using.

In a small bowl, whisk all the ingredients together and store in an airtight glass jar for up to 1 month in the pantry.

VARIATION 1 Ranch Dressing: Combine 3 tablespoons of seasoning, 1 cup of mayonnaise, and ½ cup to 1 cup dairy-free milk (depending on your desired dressing thickness). Whisk and refrigerate in an airtight glass jar for up to 1 week.

VARIATION 2 Ranch Dip: Whisk 3 tablespoons of seasoning into 1 cup of sour cream or dairy-free sour cream. Refrigerate for at least 30 minutes before serving. Serve with fresh cut vegetables or your favorite chips.

SUBSTITUTION TIP *If you eat dairy, substitute an equal amount of milk powder for the coconut milk powder.*

PER SERVING (2 tablespoons): Calories: 43; Total fat: 0g; Total carbs: 7g; Sugar: 5g; Protein: 4g; Fiber: 0g; Sodium: 384mg

Prep time: 10 minutes

Cook time: 4 hours

8 cups water

3 pounds bone-in
chicken pieces

1 small onion, halved

1 large carrot,
ends trimmed

1 celery stalk

2 garlic cloves, halved

¼ teaspoon
ground turmeric

Homemade Chicken Stock

Dairy-free · Egg-free I make this recipe in a 3-quart stockpot. If you use a smaller pot, reduce the amounts of the ingredients but add enough water to cover all of them. Avoid the temptation to embellish the recipe by adding in cabbage and all sorts of root vegetables. Cabbage can overpower the flavor, and an overabundance of root vegetables will cloud the stock. I don't salt my stock until I use it, but feel free to add up to 1 teaspoon of salt to taste. Use homemade stock in other recipes, as the cooking liquid for rice or other grains, and for making gravy.

1. Place all the ingredients in a large stockpot over high heat.

2. Add more water if needed so the chicken and vegetables are fully covered. Bring to a full boil. Cover the pot and reduce the heat to low.

3. Simmer for 4 hours. Turn off the heat and allow the stock to cool.

4. Ladle out the solids (discard or use as you wish), then strain the stock using a fine-mesh strainer or cheesecloth.

5. Refrigerate in airtight jars for up to 5 days or freeze for up to 2 months in freezer-safe containers.

VARIATION 1 **Slow Cooker Stock:** Add all the ingredients to a 6-quart slow cooker. Cover and cook on low for 8 to 10 hours.

VARIATION 2 **Pressure Cooker Stock:** Add all the ingredients to your electric pressure cooker. Be sure not to exceed the maximum fill line. Cook according to your pressure cooker's manual. I use the Soup and Stew setting. Allow the pressure to release for at least 30 minutes, if possible.

SUBSTITUTION TIPS *For vegetable stock, use about 6 cups roughly chopped vegetables in place of the chicken. You can also use this recipe to make beef or fish stock by substituting 1 pound beef and bones or 1 to 2 pounds fish bones with a small amount of meat on them for the chicken.*

PER SERVING (½ cup): Calories: 33; Total fat: 1g; Total carbs: 3g; Sugar: 0g; Protein: 3g; Fiber: 1g; Sodium: 64mg

MAKES 2 CUPS

Prep time: 5 minutes

Cook time: 5 minutes

2 cups stock

1 tablespoon unsalted butter or dairy-free butter

1 tablespoon cornstarch

1 tablespoon cold water

½ teaspoon salt

½ teaspoon dried sage

⅛ teaspoon freshly ground black pepper

Perfect Gravy Every Time

Dairy-free · *Egg-free* A ladle of gravy can make or break a fluffy scoop of mashed potatoes (or Roasted Garlic Smashed Cauliflower, page 74). Gluten-free gravy is easy to make anytime with a variety of liquids and starches. Read the full recipe and variations before you begin to make sure you select the correct starch and liquid for your gravy.

1. In a large saucepan, heat the stock and butter over medium-high heat.

2. In a small bowl, whisk together the cornstarch and cold water.

3. When the broth begins to come to a gentle boil, pour the cornstarch-water mixture into it. Whisk and bring the mixture to a full boil, then remove from heat.

4. Season with the salt, sage, and pepper.

VARIATION **Cream Gravy:** Substitute dairy or plant-based milk for the stock.

SUBSTITUTION TIP *Use 2 tablespoons of tapioca starch in place of the cornstarch. Tapioca thickens quickly and doesn't need to be boiled. Too much tapioca turns gravy to gel.*

MAKE-AHEAD TIP *If you plan to freeze the gravy, do not use the cornstarch. The gravy will lose its thickness and turn spongy. Instead, use 1 tablespoon arrowroot starch. Combine with the cold water, then whisk the mixture into the hot liquid. Stir until the gravy thickens, about 1 minute. Do not boil the gravy, as arrowroot is a low-temperature thickener. Do not use arrowroot starch with dairy products, as it turns to slime.*

PER SERVING (¼ cup): Calories: 38; Total fat: 2g; Total carbs: 3g; Sugar: 1g; Protein: 2g; Fiber: 0g; Sodium: 233mg

Prep time: 15 minutes

Cook time: 25 minutes

5
ING

232 grams (about
1½ cups) Gigi's
Everyday Gluten-Free
Flour (page 27),
plus more for dusting

2 teaspoons guar gum

¾ teaspoon
baking powder

½ teaspoon salt

4 tablespoons
palm shortening

½ cup warm
water, divided

Flour Tortillas

Vegan No cracking, no crumbling, and no cardboard-tasting tortillas here. Shortening is the key to tender, pliable tortillas. I use organic palm shortening made without hydrogenated oils and trans fats. Two additional keys to success are adding the right amount of water and not overcooking the tortillas.

1. Place the flour, guar gum, baking powder, and salt in the bowl of your stand mixer. Beat on low speed for 30 seconds.

2. Add the shortening in 4 pieces and beat on low until the mixture resembles crumbs.

3. Add ¼ cup of the water, then beat on low speed for about 1 minute. Add the remaining water 1 tablespoon at a time with the mixer running on low speed (you may not need all the water). Increase the mixer to medium-low, then to medium to form the dough. It takes a couple of minutes for the dough to come together. It should come together in a large ball but should not be sticky to the touch. If the dough is still too dry, add more water, 1 tablespoon at a time, until a ball of dough forms.

4. Using your hands, divide the dough into 8 equal portions. Place a portion between floured sheets of parchment paper and roll it to 6 inches in diameter. Repeat for each dough portion.

5. Place a skillet over high heat. Do not grease it. The pan should not be so hot that it smokes. Cook each tortilla for 2 to 3 minutes per side, until it begins to show dark spots. Do not overcook or the tortillas will be dry, hard, and will crack.

6. Transfer each tortilla to a plate and cover with a kitchen towel or aluminum foil to keep warm.

MAKE-AHEAD TIP *Prepare the tortillas through step 4, then layer the uncooked tortillas between sheets of wax paper. Wrap well and freeze for up to 1 month. Thaw at room temperature before cooking.*

PER SERVING (1 tortilla): Calories: 160; Total fat: 7g; Total carbs: 23g; Sugar: 0g; Protein: 2g; Fiber: 1g; Sodium: 154mg

Prep time: 15 minutes

Cook time: 10 minutes

300 grams (about 2 cups)
Gigi's Everyday Gluten-
Free Flour (page 27)

1 teaspoon guar gum

¼ teaspoon salt

½ cup palm shortening,
at room temperature

¼ cup dairy-free
butter, cold

¼ cup cold water

1 tablespoon apple
cider vinegar

The Only Pie Crust You'll Ever Need

Vegan Let your food processor do the work of mixing this pie crust for you. It's ready to roll right away and makes an excellent pie, quiche, or topping for Chicken Pot Pie (page 162). This dough is forgiving, so if it tears or cracks while rolling, simply pinch it back together and carry on.

1. In the bowl of your food processor, combine the flour, guar gum, and salt. Pulse a few times to blend.

2. Add the shortening and dairy-free butter. Pulse several times until coarse crumbs form.

3. Add the water and vinegar, then pulse several times. Turn on the food processor to blend the dough until it comes together in a ball. I consistently make this crust with ¼ cup water, but if your dough doesn't come together in a ball after processing, add 1 more tablespoon of water. Once the dough comes together, remove it from the processor.

4. Divide the dough in half and roll it out between 2 pieces of wax or parchment paper to your desired shape and size. Carefully transfer each to a pie plate.

5. For a baked crust (unfilled), preheat the oven to 400°F and prick the dough with a fork to prevent it from bubbling. Bake for 12 minutes, or until your desired doneness. For an unbaked crust, fill and bake as your recipe directs.

VARIATION 1 **Sweet Pastry:** Add up to 3 tablespoons of sugar to the dry ingredients in step 1.

VARIATION 2 **Cheddar Pastry:** Add ½ cup of shredded Cheddar cheese to the dry ingredients in step 1.

MAKE-AHEAD TIP *Freeze an unbaked crust in the pie plate up for to 1 month. Thaw at room temperature for 15 minutes before baking or filling.*

PER SERVING (¼ crust): Calories: 207; Total fat: 20g; Total carbs: 31g; Sugar: 0g; Protein: 2g; Fiber: 1g; Sodium: 77mg

CHAPTER 4

Morning Meals

Start your day with a delicious homemade meal. Whether you prefer a sweet or savory breakfast, there's something here to satisfy. Having staples such as Quick Baking Mix (page 26) and Flour Tortillas (page 36) on hand will help get breakfast on the table fast. You'll also find grain-free options in this chapter, as well as plenty of make-ahead dishes for busy mornings.

For recipes that use oats, I recommend gluten-free purity protocol grown oats. My favorite brands include GF Harvest, Montana Gluten Free, Glutenfreeda, Gluten-Free Prairie, Libre Naturals, MadeGood, and Glanbia Nutritionals. Oats can be a tricky ingredient, and not everyone tolerates them well. Purity protocol grown means everything from seeds . . . to equipment used to plant, harvest, and manufacture . . . to finished product is tested and confirmed gluten-free. That is the only way to be certain oats are celiac-safe.

SERVES 4

Prep time: 5 minutes

Cook time: 25 minutes

2 cups Quick Baking Mix (page 26)

1 cup unsweetened coconut milk or milk of choice

2 large eggs

½ tablespoon coconut oil or avocado oil

Fluffy Three-Ingredient Pancakes

Dairy-free · ***Vegetarian*** Slightly crispy outside, light and fluffy inside— that's how pancakes should be. If you think pancakes take too long or are difficult to make, this recipe will convince you otherwise. Before you begin, make sure you have at the ready a spoon or scoop for the batter, a spatula, and a plate for the cooked pancakes. In less than 30 minutes, you can have several stacks on the table waiting to be drizzled with maple syrup. These also freeze well if you have leftovers. For a smaller batch of pancakes, halve the recipe.

1. In a large bowl, whisk together the baking mix, milk, and eggs until the batter is smooth and thick.

2. Place a large skillet over medium-high heat and grease it with the oil. Once the skillet is very hot, but not smoking, spoon ¼-cup portions of batter onto it. Cook the pancakes, undisturbed, for 2 to 3 minutes per side, until golden brown and cooked through.

3. Transfer the pancakes to a serving plate and continue cooking until all the batter is used. Serve with your favorite toppings.

VARIATION 1 **Blueberry Pancakes:** Add 1 tablespoon of sugar and ½ teaspoon of pure vanilla extract to the batter. Gently fold in ½ cup of fresh or frozen blueberries.

VARIATION 2 **PB Chocolate Chip Pancakes:** Add 2 tablespoons of peanut (or other nut/seed) butter, 1 tablespoon of sugar, and ½ teaspoon of pure vanilla extract to the batter. Stir in ⅓ cup mini chocolate chips. To serve, spread a thin layer of peanut (or other nut/seed) butter between the pancakes, and top with maple syrup and additional chocolate chips.

MAKE-AHEAD TIP *Cook, then cool the pancakes completely in a single layer. Stack the pancakes on top of one another, inserting a piece of wax paper between each, then place in a resealable plastic bag. Freeze for up to 1 month. To serve, thaw at room temperature or microwave in 30-second increments until heated through.*

PER SERVING (2 pancakes): Calories: 320; Total fat: 7g; Total carbs: 63g; Sugar: 2g; Protein: 7g; Fiber: 1g; Sodium: 604mg

Prep time: 5 minutes

Cook time: 25 minutes

28 grams (about ¼ cup) coconut flour

30 grams (about ¼ cup) tapioca starch

1 teaspoon cream of tartar

½ teaspoon baking soda

¼ teaspoon salt

2 large eggs

½ cup dairy-free milk

½ tablespoon coconut oil or avocado oil

Grain-Free Pancakes

Dairy-free · Vegetarian The batter for these pancakes is thinner than traditional pancake batter, but they still cook up light and fluffy. The trick to keeping the batter from spreading too much in the pan is to pour it slowly. The cream of tartar and baking soda create a grain-free baking powder. Traditional baking powder contains cornstarch, which is not grain-free.

1. In a large mixing bowl, combine the flour, tapioca starch, cream of tartar, baking soda, and salt and whisk until no lumps remain.

2. Add the eggs and milk. Whisk until the batter is smooth.

3. Place a large skillet over medium-high heat and grease it with the oil. Once the skillet is very hot, but not smoking, spoon ¼-cup portions of batter onto it. Cook for 1 to 2 minutes per side.

VARIATION 1 **Spice Pancakes:** Add 1 teaspoon of ground cinnamon, ½ teaspoon of ground ginger, and ¼ teaspoon of ground nutmeg in step 1.

VARIATION 2 **Sweet Pancakes:** Add up to 2 tablespoons of pure maple syrup or honey and 1 teaspoon of pure vanilla extract in step 2.

INGREDIENT TIP *If you do not have cream of tartar handy, substitute 1½ teaspoons of baking powder for the cream of tartar and baking soda. By doing so, the pancakes will not be grain-free, but the recipe will still work the same and taste equally delicious.*

PER SERVING (3 pancakes): Calories: 405; Total fat: 13g; Total carbs: 58g; Sugar: 4g; Protein: 11g; Fiber: 11g; Sodium: 765mg

1 egg, at room temperature

½ cup milk

½ cup full-fat sour cream

3 tablespoons unsalted butter, melted

190 grams (about 1¼ cups) Quick Baking Mix (page 26)

1 tablespoon granulated white or brown sugar (optional)

½ tablespoon coconut oil or avocado oil

Belgian Waffles

Vegetarian These Belgian waffles have a crisp exterior with a light, fluffy interior. This is one of the few recipes I believe is best with dairy ingredients if you can eat them; however, the substitutes listed in the allergen tip below will yield a tasty runner-up version. The sugar can be omitted, but the waffles won't be as light or crisp. Be sure to use full-fat ingredients for best results. This recipe can be doubled easily.

1. Heat a Belgian waffle iron according to manufacturer's instructions.

2. In a large mixing bowl, whisk together the egg, milk, sour cream, and melted butter until smooth.

3. Add the baking mix and sugar (if using). Whisk until no lumps remain.

4. When the waffle iron is hot, brush or mist it with the oil. Spoon batter onto the iron. I use a generous ⅓ cup of batter for each waffle.

5. Cook the waffle according to the manufacturer's recommendations. The waffle should be cooked through and crisp and golden on the outside.

6. Transfer the waffle to a plate. Oil the iron again and continue making waffles until all the batter is used. Serve the waffles immediately with your favorite toppings.

VARIATION **Crispy Bacon-Cheddar Waffles:** Cook 6 slices of bacon until crisp. Cool the bacon, then crumble it into the waffle batter along with ½ cup of grated Cheddar cheese. Cook as directed.

ALLERGEN TIP *For dairy-free waffles, substitute with a full-fat dairy-free version of sour cream or yogurt (plain, unsweetened); a plant-based milk, like unsweetened coconut milk; and a dairy-free butter.*

PER SERVING (2 waffles): Calories: 711; Total fat: 38g; Total carbs: 82g; Sugar: 5g; Protein: 13g; Fiber: 11g; Sodium: 501mg

Prep time: 5 minutes

Cook time: 10 minutes

2 large eggs

¼ cup milk

1 teaspoon pure
vanilla extract

⅛ teaspoon salt

⅛ teaspoon
ground cinnamon

2 tablespoons coconut
oil or other high-heat-
tolerant oil, divided

4 (1-inch-thick)
slices bread

Classic French Toast

Vegetarian Making French toast is all about proportions. Use 1 egg and 2 tablespoons of milk per person. Using that math, you can make as few or as many servings as you like with this recipe. Choose sturdy, great-tasting bread, like my Top 8–Free Sandwich Bread (page 191). It holds its shape after soaking up the custard mixture, and the inside remains plush and creamy when cooked.

1. In a shallow bowl that will accommodate the bread slices (or an 8-by-8-inch baking dish), whisk together the eggs, milk, vanilla, salt, and cinnamon.

2. Heat a large skillet over medium-high heat and add 2 teaspoons of oil. While the oil heats, place 2 slices of the bread in the egg mixture. After 30 seconds, turn the bread carefully and let it soak up the egg for about 30 more seconds.

3. Lift each slice carefully, allowing excess egg mixture to drain off, and place it in the skillet. Cook for 1 to 2 minutes per side, until browned and crisp on the exterior. If you feel you need to add oil to the pan when you flip the slices, add another 1 to 2 teaspoons. Transfer to a serving plate and repeat with the remaining bread.

4. Serve the French toast hot with pure maple syrup, honey, or a dusting of confectioners sugar.

VARIATION 1 **Savory French Toast:** Omit the vanilla and cinnamon. Add ⅛ teaspoon of freshly ground black pepper. Sprinkle with finely grated Parmesan cheese after cooking, if desired.

VARIATION 2 **Banana Bread French Toast:** For next-level French toast, use slices of Quick & Easy Banana Bread (page 46). Omit the vanilla and salt, and cook as directed, being very careful with the slices so they do not break. Serve with fresh strawberries and whipped cream, if desired.

ALLERGEN TIP *Use dairy-free milk to make this recipe dairy-free.*

PER SERVING (2 pieces): Calories: 345; Total fat: 21g; Total carbs: 26g; Sugar: 5g; Protein: 13g; Fiber: 2g; Sodium: 488mg

SERVES 4

Prep time: 5 minutes

Cook time: 20 minutes

¼ teaspoon coconut oil or avocado oil

160 grams (about 2 cups) purity protocol oats

1½ cups unsweetened coconut milk (from a carton, not a can)

½ cup dried, unsweetened coconut flakes

1 large egg

2 tablespoons pure maple syrup or honey

1 tablespoon coconut oil or dairy-free butter, melted

2 teaspoons pure vanilla extract

1 teaspoon baking powder

½ teaspoon salt

⅓ cup dark chocolate chips, divided

Healthy Coconut-Chocolate Baked Oatmeal

Dairy-free · Vegetarian This is the easiest breakfast you'll ever make! Mix everything in the baking dish and in about 20 minutes, you'll be spooning up bowls of warm-from-the-oven oatmeal reminiscent of a chocolate-covered coconut candy bar. The best news is, this oatmeal is much healthier and will keep you feeling satisfied until lunchtime. Use 70 percent (or higher) dark chocolate for an antioxidant boost.

1. Preheat the oven to 350°F. Lightly grease an 8-by-8-inch baking dish with the oil.

2. Put the oats, coconut milk, coconut flakes, egg, maple syrup, coconut oil, vanilla, baking powder, and salt in the baking dish. Stir to blend, making sure the egg is fully scrambled and incorporated.

3. Stir in ¼ cup of chocolate chips. Bake for 20 minutes.

4. Top the baked oatmeal with the remaining chocolate chips and serve warm. Refrigerate leftovers in an airtight container for up to 3 days.

VARIATION **PB&J Baked Oatmeal:** Omit the coconut flakes, maple syrup, coconut oil, and chocolate chips. Add ½ cup of warm peanut butter or other nut or seed butter. Before baking, top the oatmeal with teaspoons of your favorite jam, about ¼ cup total.

MAKE-AHEAD TIP *Double the recipe and prepare in a 9-by-13-inch baking pan. Cool completely in the pan, then portion the baked oatmeal into individual serving containers. Seal and freeze for up to 1 month.*

PER SERVING Calories: 397; Total fat: 26g; Total carbs: 35g; Sugar: 14g; Protein: 7g; Fiber: 6g; Sodium: 367mg

Prep time: 5 minutes

Cook time: 5 minutes

½ cup unsweetened applesauce

3 tablespoons sunflower seeds, toasted and ground

2 tablespoons ground flaxseed

2 tablespoons chia seeds

2 tablespoons unsweetened toasted coconut flakes

2 tablespoons coconut cream

2 Medjool dates, pitted and chopped

1 teaspoon ground cinnamon, plus more for serving (optional)

⅛ teaspoon salt

Grain-Free Breakfast Porridge

Vegan If you miss eating warm cereal for breakfast, this is a satisfying substitute. It is unique in the grain-free category because it is also nut-free. It is hearty and satisfying, sweet and savory, and cooks up quick enough that there's no reason not to start your day with a solid breakfast.

1. In a small saucepan over medium heat, combine all the ingredients. Stir to blend as the mixture heats.

2. Heat until just bubbling (do not boil), then remove from heat. Serve immediately, topped with a dash of cinnamon, if desired.

VARIATION **Pumpkin Porridge:** Substitute pumpkin purée for the applesauce. Add a dash of nutmeg.

INGREDIENT TIP *Substitute heavy (whipping) cream for the coconut cream and nuts for the sunflower seeds.*

PER SERVING Calories: 634; Total fat: 40g; Total carbs: 68g; Sugar: 45g; Protein: 12g; Fiber: 17g; Sodium: 888mg

Prep time: 10 minutes

Cook time: 40 minutes

¼ cup sunflower oil, plus ¼ teaspoon

3 small to medium ripe bananas

½ cup unsweetened applesauce

2 large eggs

¼ cup pure maple syrup

2 teaspoons pure vanilla extract

240 grams (about 1½ cups) Gigi's Everyday Gluten-Free Flour (page 27)

1 teaspoon baking powder

½ teaspoon baking soda

½ teaspoon salt

1 teaspoon ground cinnamon (optional)

Quick & Easy Banana Bread

Dairy-free • *Vegetarian* Blending very ripe bananas with a mixer is one of my favorite tips for making the best banana bread. This ensures no soggy chunks of banana in the bread and creates a smooth, easily sliceable loaf. The unsweetened applesauce and a bit of oil keep this bread moist enough to enjoy for several days without a need to reheat it.

1. Preheat the oven to 350°F. Grease a metal 9-by-5-inch loaf pan with ¼ teaspoon of oil.

2. In the bowl of your stand mixer, beat the remaining oil, bananas, applesauce, eggs, maple syrup, and vanilla until mostly smooth, about 1 minute.

3. With the mixer off, add the flour, baking powder, baking soda, salt, and cinnamon (if using). Mix at low speed for 30 seconds, then increase to medium until the dry ingredients are fully incorporated. Scrape down the sides and bottom of the bowl, if needed.

4. Pour the batter into the loaf pan. Bake for about 40 minutes. The loaf will rise to a domed center, and cracks will appear on top of the loaf. The center will be set and will spring back when lightly pressed.

5. Let the loaf cool almost completely before removing it from the pan and slicing.

VARIATION 1 **Chocolate Chip Banana Bread:** Stir ½ cup of chocolate chips into the batter after mixing in the dry ingredients. Sprinkle a few chocolate chips on top of the batter before baking.

VARIATION 2 **Pumpkin Banana Bread:** Replace the applesauce with the same amount of pumpkin purée, and add 2 teaspoons of ground cinnamon and ½ teaspoon of nutmeg.

INGREDIENT TIP *Peel and freeze ripe bananas for up to 1 month. To use, thaw at room temperature or microwave in 15-second intervals until soft.*

PER SERVING (1 slice): Calories: 160; Total fat: 6g; Total carbs: 25g; Sugar: 9g; Protein: 2g; Fiber: 3g; Sodium: 210mg

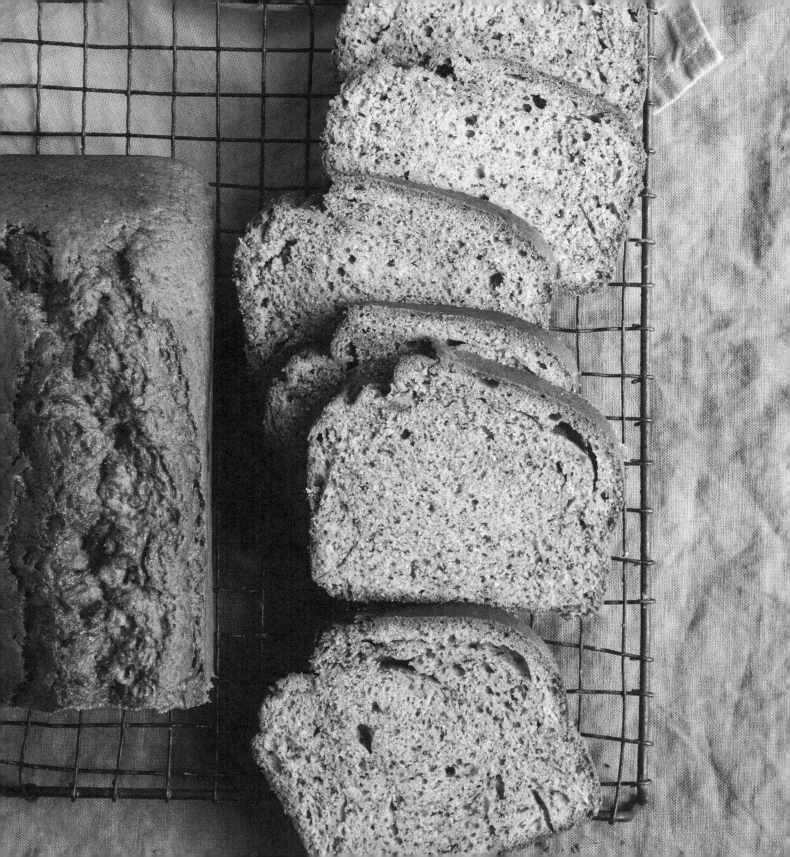

Prep time: 10 minutes

Cook time: 20 minutes

300 grams (about
2 cups) Quick Baking
Mix (page 26)

¼ cup palm shortening

1 large egg

½ cup dairy-free milk

½ tablespoon dairy-free
butter, melted

½ tablespoon
sugar (optional)

Classic Scones

Dairy-free • Vegetarian If you love Southern biscuits, chances are you love scones, too. The difference between them is that scones contain egg and biscuits do not. Some scones, like this recipe, have a little sugar, too. Use this recipe as a blank canvas for customizing scones to your tastes by adding up to ½ cup of dried fruit, nuts, or even chocolate chips.

1. Preheat the oven to 425°F. Line a baking sheet with parchment paper or grease it lightly with oil or butter.

2. Place the baking mix and shortening in a medium bowl. Use a fork to cut the shortening into the baking mix until the mixture resembles coarse crumbs.

3. Add the egg and milk and stir until a dough forms.

4. Place the dough on the prepared baking sheet and pat it into a circle about 7 inches across and ¾ inch thick.

5. Use a sharp knife to score the circle of dough into 8 sections, but do not cut through the dough.

6. Brush the dough with the melted butter and sprinkle with the sugar (if using).

7. Bake for 20 minutes, or until the top appears dry and the scone is baked through. You will see cracks around the outer edges of the dough.

8. Remove the scones from the oven and let them cool on the baking sheet for 20 minutes before cutting into 8 wedges. Serve with butter and jam.

VARIATION **Sun-Dried Tomato Scones:** Omit the sugar and add ¼ cup of drained and chopped sun-dried tomatoes and ¼ cup of shredded Parmesan or Asiago cheese.

SUBSTITUTION TIP *If you eat dairy ingredients, feel free to use regular milk and butter.*

PER SERVING (1 scone): Calories: 240; Total fat: 13g; Total carbs: 32g; Sugar: 2g; Protein: 3g; Fiber: 1g; Sodium: 286mg

MAKES 12 MUFFINS

Prep time: 10 minutes

Cook time: 20 minutes

30
MIN

¼ teaspoon coconut oil or avocado oil

80 grams (about 1 cup) purity protocol oats

155 grams (about 1 cup) Gigi's Everyday Gluten-Free Flour (page 27)

½ cup coconut sugar

1 tablespoon baking powder

½ teaspoon salt

½ cup no-added-sugar sunflower seed butter

1¼ cups unsweetened coconut milk

2 teaspoons pure vanilla extract

⅓ cup chocolate chips, plus more for topping (optional)

Sunflower Seed Butter Muffins

Vegan I turn to this recipe often. My daughter loves these muffins for breakfast with a glass of coconut milk, and my husband takes them to work for a mid-morning snack. While I use sunflower seed butter in the recipe, feel free to substitute it with any nut butter or seed butter to keep the muffins dairy-free. One tip: Measure the oats *before* pulsing them in the food processor. If you process before measuring, the quantity will exceed what is called for and your muffins will be dry.

1. Preheat the oven to 375°F. Lightly grease a 12-cup muffin tin with the oil or line the cups with parchment liners.

2. Place the oats in the bowl of a food processor and pulse until they resemble a coarse flour.

3. In a large mixing bowl, combine the ground oats, flour, sugar, baking powder, and salt. Whisk to blend.

4. Add the sunflower seed butter, coconut milk, and vanilla. Stir to combine. Stir in the chocolate chips.

5. Divide the batter evenly between the muffin cups. Sprinkle the tops with a few additional chocolate chips, if desired.

6. Bake for 20 minutes, or until the centers spring back when gently pressed. Cool completely before serving.

VARIATION **Raisin Spice Muffins:** Add 1 teaspoon of ground cinnamon, ½ teaspoon of ground ginger, ¼ teaspoon of ground nutmeg, and ½ cup of raisins. Omit the chocolate chips.

SUBSTITUTION TIP *You can use brown sugar in place of the coconut sugar; however, I recommend reducing the amount to ⅓ cup.*

PER SERVING (1 muffin): Calories: 175; Total fat: 7g; Total carbs: 25g; Sugar: 12g; Protein: 4g; Fiber: 2g; Sodium: 153mg

Prep time: 5 minutes

Cook time: 5 minutes

4 large eggs

¼ teaspoon salt

1 tablespoon
unsalted butter

Freshly ground black
pepper (optional)

Snipped chives (optional)

Perfect Scrambled Eggs

Vegetarian Perfect scrambled eggs rely on technique and timing. First, spend a full 90 seconds whisking your eggs into fluffy submission. Second, remove them from the pan before they are fully cooked. If you're tempted to add milk or cream to the whisked eggs, don't. Additional liquid causes the eggs to separate and dry out.

1. In a medium bowl, whisk the eggs and salt together for 90 seconds.

2. In a medium skillet, melt the butter over medium heat. Swirl the butter around to coat the skillet surface, then pour in the eggs. Allow them to set for 20 to 30 seconds, then very gently use a spatula to push the eggs from the edges of the skillet toward the center of the pan in wide ribbons. Use the spatula to turn the eggs and cook until just shy of cooked through. Turn off the heat and spoon the eggs onto serving plates.

3. Top the eggs with black pepper and a pinch of chives (if using). Serve immediately.

VARIATION 1 **Goat Cheese Eggs:** After adding the eggs to the skillet, top with 2 tablespoons of goat cheese crumbles.

VARIATION 2 **Avocado-Tomato Eggs:** After plating, top each serving with ½ small diced avocado and 2 tablespoons diced tomato. Add a pinch of additional salt on top.

PER SERVING Calories: 193; Total fat: 15g; Total carbs: 1g; Sugar: 1g; Protein: 13g; Fiber: 0g; Sodium: 431mg

SERVES 6

Prep time: 10 minutes

Cook time: 15 minutes

¼ teaspoon coconut oil or avocado oil

3 medium carrots, ends trimmed

½ red bell pepper

8 large eggs

½ cup fresh cilantro or flat-leaf parsley

½ teaspoon salt

¼ teaspoon garlic powder

Freshly ground black pepper

Mini Frittatas

Dairy-free • *Vegetarian* This is my favorite make-ahead quick and healthy breakfast. Anyone who loves eggs will enjoy this revamped way to serve them. Feel free to switch up the veggies and use whatever is in season. Try asparagus in the spring and shredded sweet potatoes in the fall. Adjust the seasonings to suit your tastes and create your own custom frittatas.

1. Preheat the oven to 350°F. Grease a 12-cup muffin tin with the oil.

2. Cut the carrots and pepper into chunks, and transfer them to the bowl of a food processor; pulse into small pieces. Alternatively, finely chop the pepper by hand and grate the carrots.

3. In a large bowl, whisk the eggs (or use an immersion blender to blend the eggs quickly). Stir in the chopped vegetables and the cilantro, salt, garlic powder, and black pepper.

4. Divide the mixture evenly between the muffin cups. Bake for about 15 minutes. The frittatas will puff up as they bake and deflate slightly as they cool.

5. Serve immediately, or let the frittatas cool to room temperature, then refrigerate in an airtight container for up to 3 days.

VARIATION 1 **Cheese Eggs:** Omit the vegetables and add 1 cup shredded cheese to the eggs.

VARIATION 2 **Pancetta Frittata Cups:** Place a thin slice of pancetta in each muffin cup, spreading it out to fit the cup, then fill with the egg mixture.

PER SERVING (2 frittatas): Calories: 113; Total fat: 7g; Total carbs: 4g; Sugar: 3g; Protein: 9g; Fiber: 1g; Sodium: 309mg

Prep time: 5 minutes

Cook time: 15 minutes

ING MIN POT

1 teaspoon coconut oil

2 large sweet potatoes

1 teaspoon fennel seeds

4 large eggs

½ teaspoon salt

Sheet Pan Eggs in Sweet Potato Nests

Dairy-free · Vegetarian Spiral-cut sweet potatoes, seasoned with salt and fennel, hold eggs in place while they bake to delicate perfection. This is a fun breakfast for Easter morning or for any spring brunch!

1. Preheat the oven to 375°F. Grease a large rimmed baking sheet with the oil.

2. Wash, peel, and spiral-cut the sweet potatoes. You need about 1 cup of spirals for each nest.

3. Place 1-cup portions of spiral-cut sweet potatoes on the baking sheet, spacing them a few inches apart. Shape the spirals into nests and form an opening in the center 1½ to 2 inches in diameter. Sprinkle with the fennel seeds.

4. Crack an egg into each nest. Sprinkle each nest and egg with the salt.

5. Bake for about 12 minutes for a soft-centered egg with a slightly runny yolk. If you like your eggs cooked more, bake for another 2 or 3 minutes.

6. Carefully transfer the nests to serving plates. Serve immediately.

VARIATION **Sheet Pan Eggs in Hash Brown Nests:** Use regular potatoes for a hash brown–style nest.

INGREDIENT TIP *If you don't have a spiral slicer, you can use a vegetable peeler to cut the sweet potatoes into thin ribbons. The "nest" effect will be lost, but the dish will be just as delicious.*

MAKE-AHEAD TIP *Make nests (through step 3) up to 2 hours ahead of time, and refrigerate on the baking sheet until ready to add the eggs and bake.*

PER SERVING Calories: 144; Total fat: 6g; Total carbs: 15g; Sugar: 0g; Protein: 7g; Fiber: 2g; Sodium: 361mg

SERVES 6

Prep time: 10 minutes

Cook time: 50 minutes

1 POT

¼ teaspoon coconut oil or avocado oil

5 cups peeled and grated potatoes

½ cup diced onion

½ cup diced celery

2 cups shredded Monterey Jack cheese or dairy-free cheese

¼ cup melted unsalted butter or dairy-free butter, or ghee

1 teaspoon salt

1 teaspoon garlic powder

⅛ teaspoon freshly ground black pepper

1 cup milk or dairy-free milk of your choice

½ teaspoon dried parsley (optional)

6 large eggs

Hash Brown Casserole with Nested Eggs

Dairy-free · Vegetarian This casserole needs to be at your next brunch! It's so easy to put together—all the ingredients go straight into the casserole dish, so there's minimal cleanup. The nested eggs add pizzazz, so it's sure to impress any guest. It makes terrific leftovers, too. Simply cool, portion into storage containers, and refrigerate for a hearty breakfast any day of the week.

1. Preheat the oven to 375°F. Lightly grease a 3-quart casserole dish with the oil.

2. Place the potatoes in the casserole dish and evenly sprinkle the onion, celery, and cheese over the top. Drizzle the butter or ghee over the top, then evenly sprinkle on the salt, garlic powder, and pepper. Pour the milk evenly over the top. Sprinkle with the parsley (if using).

3. Bake for 45 minutes. Use a spoon to carefully create 6 round openings in the hash browns. Crack an egg into each of the 6 openings so that the eggs are nested in the casserole.

4. Bake for 5 minutes for eggs with a soft center, or a few minutes longer if you prefer your eggs cooked completely through. Serve hot.

VARIATION **Country-Style Hash Browns:** Prepare as directed and add ½ pound of cooked and crumbled breakfast sausage, 1 cup of sliced mushrooms, and ½ cup of diced green bell pepper to the potato mixture (layering as with the other ingredients), and top with an additional 1 cup of cheese. Omit the eggs and bake for 45 minutes.

SUBSTITUTION TIP *Substitute a 1-pound bag of frozen hash brown–style potatoes instead of grating your own. Look for brands with grated potatoes as the only ingredient.*

PER SERVING Calories: 236; Total fat: 16g; Total carbs: 13g; Sugar: 3g; Protein: 10g; Fiber: 2g; Sodium: 559mg

SERVES 10

Prep time: 15 minutes

Cook time: 45 minutes

¼ teaspoon coconut oil or avocado oil

2 pounds breakfast sausage

1 cup diced sweet onion

½ cup shredded carrot

½ cup diced celery

2 garlic cloves, minced

2 cups shredded sweet potato

2 cups shredded white Cheddar cheese or dairy-free cheese

1 cup Quick Baking Mix (page 26)

2 cups milk or unsweetened coconut milk

4 large eggs

Breakfast Casserole

This is my family's most requested breakfast. Thank goodness it's easy to make! Hands-on time is short, and I can tidy up the kitchen while it bakes. That makes this dish especially well-suited for holidays and brunch gatherings. It can feed a crowd, but if you have leftovers, they freeze well, so it's ideal to make ahead for breakfast anytime. I prefer to use sausage that's free from nitrates and nitrites.

1. Preheat the oven to 375°F. Grease a 9-by-13-inch glass baking dish with the oil.

2. In a large skillet over medium-high heat, cook the sausage, onion, carrot, and celery together until the sausage is nearly cooked through and the vegetables are tender, about 10 minutes. Add the garlic and cook 1 minute more. Transfer the mixture to the baking dish. Stir in the sweet potato and sprinkle the cheese on top. Set aside.

3. In a large bowl, combine the baking mix, milk, and eggs, and whisk until smooth. Pour this over the sausage mixture.

4. Bake for 45 minutes, or until set and cooked through.

5. Cool for 10 to 15 minutes before slicing into squares to serve.

VARIATION 1 **Meatless Breakfast Casserole:** Substitute the sausage with a meat-free "sausage" product.

VARIATION 2 **Southwest Breakfast Bake:** Substitute ½ cup of whole kernel corn for the carrot and ½ cup of black beans for the celery. Use shredded pepper jack cheese for the Cheddar. Serve with guacamole and cilantro.

PER SERVING Calories: 460; Total fat: 29g; Total carbs: 24g; Sugar: 6g; Protein: 26g; Fiber: 3g; Sodium: 997mg

SERVES 4

Prep time: 15 minutes

Cook time: 15 minutes

 MIN

Perfect Scrambled Eggs (page 50), made with 6 large eggs

½ tablespoon unsalted butter or dairy-free butter

4 Flour Tortillas (page 36)

½ cup shredded Cheddar cheese or dairy-free cheese

1 small tomato, diced

1 small avocado, diced

1 tablespoon thinly sliced scallions

Chopped fresh cilantro (optional)

Breakfast Burritos

Dairy-free · ***Vegetarian*** The only problem I have with these breakfast burritos is overfilling mine. They are so good that I want to put a little bit of everything in there. These are filling enough for a hearty breakfast, and they are easy to wrap in aluminum foil and take along for lunch. Cool the eggs before assembling the burritos to prevent the whole thing from becoming soggy.

1. Scramble the eggs according to the recipe, adding ½ tablespoon extra butter to accommodate the additional 2 eggs called for here. Place the cooked eggs on a plate to cool for 10 minutes before assembling the burritos.

2. Place the tortillas on a flat work surface. Divide the cheese between the centers of each tortilla, then top each with the eggs, dividing evenly.

3. Top with the tomato, avocado, scallions, and cilantro (if using). To roll the burritos, fold up the bottom of each tortilla and tuck in the sides over the filling. With both ends tightly in place, place the burritos on individual plates, seam-side down.

VARIATION 1 **Egg Salad Wraps:** Wrap egg salad and romaine lettuce in tortillas.

VARIATION 2 **Pan-Grilled Burritos:** Fill the burritos as desired and cook them over medium-high heat in a lightly greased skillet until brown and crisp on the outside.

PER SERVING Calories: 336; Total fat: 24g; Total carbs: 17g; Sugar: 2g; Protein: 16g; Fiber: 5g; Sodium: 208mg

CHAPTER 5

Small Bites & Snacks

Making your own snacks means you know exactly what you're eating. Instead of packaged chips or cookies, whip up a quick batch of Ultimate Guacamole (page 58) or Pimiento Cheese Spread (page 61) and dig in with fresh veggies. Whole foods and healthy fats have staying power and keep you feeling full longer than store-bought, empty-calorie temptations.

Many of these recipes translate well into appetizers. Pair Traditional Deviled Eggs (page 62) with Smoked Salmon Roll-Ups (page 64), Persian-Spiced Carrot Hummus (page 60), and Salted Fennel Crackers (page 184) and you have a party! Or make one of my daughter's favorite lunches by spreading pimiento cheese between Flour Tortillas (page 36) and making a quesadilla.

If you need a sweet bite, I tucked in some treats that are nutrient-dense enough for snack time but free of refined sugar. They are great to make ahead of time and freeze for whenever a snack attack hits.

4 ripe avocados, halved, pitted, and peeled, divided

Juice of 1 lime

Zest of 1 lime

1 medium tomato, peeled, seeded, cored, and finely diced

1 small sweet onion, finely diced (about ⅓ cup)

⅓ cup green olives, pitted and diced

¼ cup chopped fresh cilantro

2 tablespoons minced fresh chives

1 garlic clove, finely minced

1 to 2 teaspoons minced fresh jalapeño pepper (optional)

1 teaspoon ground cumin

¼ teaspoon salt

Ultimate Guacamole

Vegan This is my all-time-favorite guacamole recipe. It's loaded with flavor, texture, and color. While I love it as a dip for fresh vegetables or tortilla chips, my favorite way to eat it is as a sandwich spread with roasted red peppers, sprouts, and whatever other veggies I have on hand.

1. On a large plate or shallow bowl with sides at least 2 inches deep, mash 2 avocados. Chop the remaining 2 avocados and add them to the plate. Drizzle the lime juice on top.

2. Add the lime zest, tomato, onion, olives, cilantro, chives, garlic, jalapeño, cumin, and salt, and stir until everything is incorporated.

VARIATION 1 **Spicy Bacon Guac:** Add 4 crumbled strips of crispy cooked bacon and ¼ teaspoon of red pepper flakes.

VARIATION 2 **Cheesy Southwestern Guac:** Spread the guacamole in a serving bowl. Top with ½ cup of drained cooked black beans, ½ cup of roasted corn kernels, and ½ cup of crumbled goat cheese.

PER SERVING Calories: 292; Total fat: 27g; Total carbs: 14g; Sugar: 2g; Protein: 3g; Fiber: 10g; Sodium: 168mg

Prep time: 15 minutes

30
MIN

1 tablespoon
extra-virgin olive oil

1 teaspoon
balsamic vinegar

1 large avocado, halved,
pitted, and peeled

¼ teaspoon salt, divided

Pinch red pepper flakes

2 thick slices Top 8–Free
Sandwich Bread
(page 191)

2 teaspoons
unsalted butter or
dairy-free butter

½ cup fresh salad greens

Avocado Toast

Dairy-free · ***Egg-free*** · ***Vegan*** Avocado toast is everywhere these days, but the best I ever had was at a café in Paris a few years ago. The bread was freshly baked and thickly sliced, toasted perfectly, loaded with a seasoned chunky avocado mash, topped with microgreens, and drizzled with balsamic dressing. I make my own version using thick slices of homemade bread and enjoy it as a delicious snack or light lunch.

1. In a small bowl, whisk together the oil and balsamic vinegar. Set aside.

2. In a medium bowl, mash half the avocado. Dice the other half and stir into the mashed. Add salt to taste and a pinch of red pepper flakes. Set aside.

3. Toast the bread to your liking. Spread each slice with 1 teaspoon of butter and sprinkle each with the remaining salt.

4. Divide the avocado mixture between the toasts, then top each with the greens. Drizzle the dressing over the top. Serve immediately.

VARIATION 1 **White Bean Toast:** Substitute ¾ cup of cooked white beans for the avocado.

VARIATION 2 **BLTA Toast:** For an open-faced sandwich, add 2 slices of crisp bacon and a large slice of tomato to each toast.

INGREDIENT TIP *Bread that is just past its prime and has started to dry out a bit makes the best toast.*

PER SERVING Calories: 370; Total fat: 31g; Total carbs: 20g; Sugar: 2g; Protein: 6g; Fiber: 9g; Sodium: 720mg

Prep time: 10 minutes

Cook time: 25 minutes

1 pound carrots

5 garlic cloves, unpeeled

¼ cup tahini

2 tablespoons
extra-virgin olive oil

1 tablespoon freshly
squeezed lemon juice

1 teaspoon dried cilantro

½ teaspoon
ground cumin

½ teaspoon
ground turmeric

½ teaspoon salt

⅛ teaspoon red
pepper flakes

Persian-Spiced Carrot Hummus

Vegan This recipe uses foundational flavors of Persian cooking without the need to buy a specialty spice blend. Cook the carrots first, then let them cool while you gather the other ingredients. A quick spin in the food processor turns out a creamy, bean-free hummus with an exotic flavor.

1. Preheat the oven to 425°F. Line a roasting pan with aluminum foil.

2. Place the carrots and garlic cloves in the pan and roast for 20 to 25 minutes, until the carrots are tender.

3. When the garlic is cool enough to handle, squeeze the garlic from each clove into the bowl of a food processor. Add the carrots, tahini, olive oil, lemon juice, cilantro, cumin, turmeric, salt, and red pepper flakes. Process until the hummus is smooth. You will need to turn off the processor and scrape down the sides of the bowl a couple of times so that everything blends well.

4. Spoon into a serving dish and serve with Salted Fennel Crackers (page 184) or Versatile Flatbread (page 194), or use as a sandwich spread.

VARIATION **Persian-Spiced Sweet Potato Hummus:** Substitute about 2 cups mashed sweet potato for the carrots.

PER SERVING Calories: 102; Total fat: 8g; Total carbs: 8g; Sugar: 3g; Protein: 2g; Fiber: 2g; Sodium: 196mg

SERVES 12

Prep time: 20 minutes

COOK ING MIN

1 (4-ounce) jar diced pimiento peppers, well-drained

8 ounces cream cheese, at room temperature

2 cups freshly grated sharp Cheddar cheese, divided

⅓ cup mayonnaise

½ teaspoon garlic powder

½ teaspoon salt

Pimiento Cheese Spread

Vegetarian Take time to grate your own Cheddar. It makes a significant difference in how this classic Southern sandwich spread tastes. I put the cream cheese on the counter to soften while I grate the cheese. You can certainly stir the mixture by hand, but I prefer the whipped texture I get by using the food processor.

1. Measure out 1 tablespoon of the pimiento peppers and set it aside.

2. In the bowl of a food processor, combine the rest of the pimiento peppers, the cream cheese, 1 cup of Cheddar cheese, the mayonnaise, garlic powder, and salt. Pulse several times until the ingredients start to come together.

3. Turn off the processor and scrape down the sides of the bowl, then process again until the mixture is smooth. This spread is very stiff and thick, as it should be, but if you prefer it thinner, use a tablespoon or two of milk to thin it to your liking.

4. Transfer the spread to a bowl and stir in the remaining cup of cheese and the reserved tablespoon of pimientos. Serve immediately or chill before serving.

5. Refrigerate in an airtight container for up to 4 days.

VARIATION 1 **Spicy Pimiento Cheese:** Stir 1 tablespoon of minced jalapeño pepper into the spread in step 4.

VARIATION 2 **Bacon Pimiento Cheese:** After blending the pimiento cheese, spoon it into a serving bowl and stir in 6 crumbled strips of crispy cooked bacon.

PER SERVING Calories: 181; Total fat: 13g; Total carbs: 4g; Sugar: 1g; Protein: 6g; Fiber: 0g; Sodium: 376mg

Prep time: 25 minutes, plus at least 30 minutes to chill

5
ING

6 large eggs

¼ cup mayonnaise

2 teaspoons yellow mustard

½ teaspoon salt

⅛ teaspoon freshly ground black pepper

Paprika, for garnish

Finely chopped fresh herbs, such as chives or parsley, for garnish

Traditional Deviled Eggs

Dairy-free • ***Vegetarian*** If you eat eggs, deviled eggs may be the perfect snack. They are protein-rich and that, combined with their fat content, helps keeps hunger at bay for hours. I keep peeled hard-boiled eggs in the refrigerator so I can whip up deviled eggs in just a few minutes.

1. Place the eggs in a 2-quart saucepan and add enough water to cover them by 1 inch. Place the pan over high heat, cover, and bring the water to a boil. As soon as the water boils, turn off the heat and let the eggs sit for 12 minutes.

2. Carefully drain the water from the saucepan and rinse the eggs in cold water for about 1 minute, until cool enough to handle. Peel the eggs under a gentle stream of cold running water, pat dry, and cut each in half lengthwise. Set aside until completely cool.

3. Once the eggs are cooled, remove the yolks and place them in a small bowl. Add the mayonnaise, mustard, salt, and pepper. Using a fork, mash the yolks to create a smooth mixture.

4. Spoon or pipe the filling into the egg whites. To pipe, use a piping bag fitted with a large open star tip, such as Wilton 4B. Garnish with the paprika and fresh herbs. Cover and chill for at least 30 minutes before serving.

VARIATION **Hummus Deviled Eggs:** Substitute hummus for the mayonnaise.

INGREDIENT TIP *Peel the eggs just after they've cooled slightly, so the shells slip off easily. If you wait until the eggs cool completely, they're nearly impossible to peel.*

PER SERVING (2 halves): Calories: 111; Total fat: 8g; Total carbs: 3g; Sugar: 1g; Protein: 7g; Fiber: 0g; Sodium: 352mg

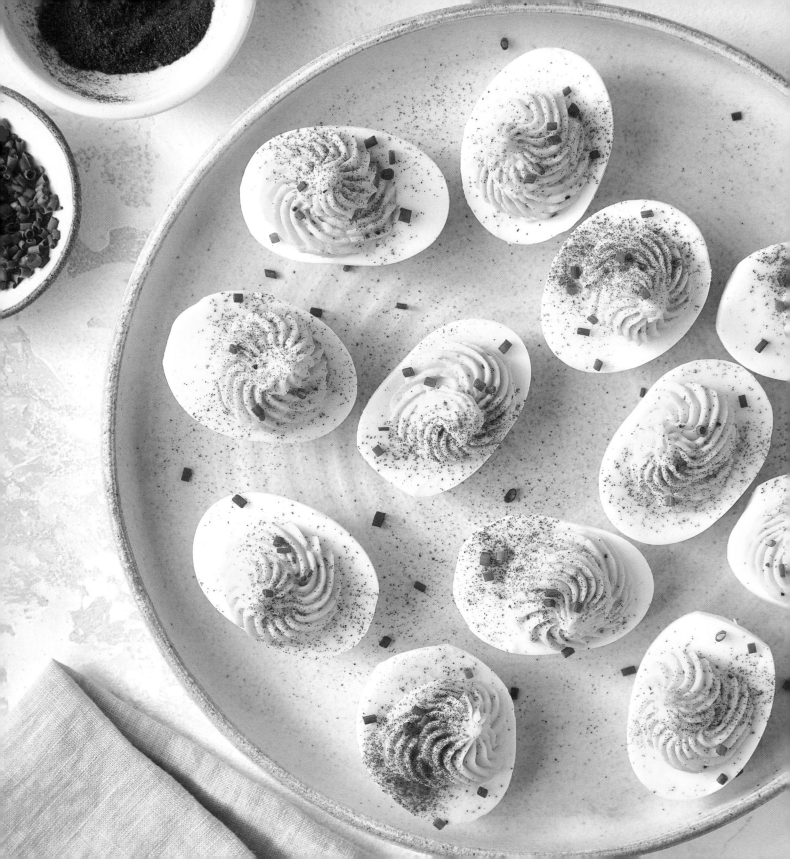

NO COOK | 30 MIN

2 ounces cream cheese,
at room temperature

1 tablespoon freshly
squeezed lemon juice

2 teaspoons grated
lemon zest

2 teaspoons dried dill

1 teaspoon
chopped capers

4 ounces thinly sliced
smoked salmon

Smoked Salmon Roll-Ups

Egg-free Smoked salmon is one of my favorite lunches. Adding a zesty cream cheese filling makes it even tastier. You can take these rolls one step further and wrap each one in a large lettuce leaf. It provides an added crunch and offsets the saltiness of the salmon.

1. In a small bowl, combine the cream cheese, lemon juice, lemon zest, dill, and capers. Stir until the mixture is smooth. Set aside.

2. Place 2 pieces of smoked salmon, overlapping, on a serving plate. Top with half the cream cheese mixture and evenly spread it over the salmon. Starting with the long edge, roll up the salmon to encase the filling. Once rolled up completely, slice it in half. Repeat with the remaining salmon and cheese filling. Serve immediately.

VARIATION **Cucumber Roll-Ups:** Instead of smoked salmon, substitute long, thin slices of cucumber. Spread with the cream cheese mixture, then roll up.

PER SERVING Calories: 171; Total fat: 13g; Total carbs: 2g; Sugar: 0g; Protein: 13g; Fiber: 0g; Sodium: 1264mg

Prep time: 10 minutes

**FOR THE
DIPPING SAUCE**

1 tablespoon Homemade
Ranch Seasoning
(page 33)

1 tablespoon
mayonnaise

1 tablespoon
Dijon mustard

1 ounce cream cheese or
dairy-free cream cheese,
at room temperature

1 tablespoon dill
pickle juice

FOR THE WRAPS

8 slices (about 6 ounces)
turkey or chicken
deli meat

1 avocado, sliced

¼ cup thinly
sliced cucumber

¼ cup thinly sliced
red onion

¼ cup red bell
pepper strips

Dill pickle slices,
for serving

Easy Deli Wraps with Dipping Sauce

Dairy-free Use high-quality deli meat that is free from preservatives and fillers. I like making these with organic roast chicken or turkey, but the roast beef variation is delicious, too. Customize your wraps with whatever suits your tastes, or whatever you have on hand in the refrigerator.

TO MAKE THE DIPPING SAUCE

In a small bowl, combine all the ingredients and stir until smooth. Set aside.

TO MAKE THE WRAPS

1. Place 2 slices of deli meat on a plate. Top with one-quarter each of the avocado, cucumber, onion, and pepper. Roll and secure with a toothpick. Repeat for a total of 4 wraps.

2. Serve with the dipping sauce and dill pickle slices.

VARIATION 1 **Roast Beef and Swiss Wraps:** Use roast beef instead of turkey or chicken. Omit the avocado, cucumber, and red pepper. Add a thin slice of Swiss cheese and thinly sliced tomato to each wrap. Omit the dipping sauce and drizzle each wrap with a small amount of prepared horseradish sauce.

VARIATION 2 **Tortilla Wraps:** Use Flour Tortillas (page 36) to encase the deli meat and fillings.

PER SERVING (2 wraps): Calories: 385; Total fat: 29g; Total carbs: 17g; Sugar: 7g; Protein: 19g; Fiber: 7g; Sodium: 845mg

SERVES 1

Prep time: 5 minutes

Cook time: 5 minutes

2 Flour Tortillas (page 36)

3 slices fresh
mozzarella cheese

3 slices tomato

3 fresh basil leaves

Salt

Freshly ground
black pepper

1 teaspoon
extra-virgin olive oil

½ teaspoon
balsamic vinegar

Caprese Quesadilla

Egg-free · *Vegetarian* I combined two of my daughter's favorite foods—Caprese salad and quesadillas—to make this delicious snack. You can easily turn this into lunch by adding a green salad on the side or by making the Chicken Caprese variation.

1. Place a skillet over medium-high heat. Add one tortilla to the skillet, then layer it with the mozzarella, tomato, and basil. Sprinkle with salt and pepper, then top with the second tortilla.

2. Cook for 2 to 3 minutes, then carefully flip the quesadilla and cook for 2 to 3 minutes more. Transfer to a serving plate and cut into 4 wedges.

3. In a small bowl, whisk together the olive oil and balsamic vinegar. Drizzle over the quesadilla and serve.

VARIATION **Chicken Caprese Quesadilla:** Add 2 ounces of thinly sliced cooked chicken breast along with the cheese and tomato.

ALLERGEN TIP *If you do not eat dairy, swap in your favorite dairy-free cheese for the mozzarella.*

PER SERVING Calories: 394; Total fat: 21g; Total carbs: 26g; Sugar: 2g; Protein: 27g; Fiber: 4g; Sodium: 689mg

MAKES 16 BITES

Prep time: 15 minutes

NO | 5 | 30
COOK | ING | MIN

10 Medjool dates, pitted

4 tablespoons toasted, salted pumpkin seeds

2 tablespoons unsweetened baking cocoa

4 tablespoons dark chocolate chips, divided

2 teaspoons pure vanilla extract

Nutritious Double-Chocolate Bites

Dairy-free • Egg-free • Vegan Although dates are high in sugar, they are relatively low on the glycemic index and do not affect blood sugar like granulated sugar does. Another bonus is their high fiber, vitamin, and mineral content. I use Lily's™ Dark Chocolate Premium Baking Chips, which have no added sugar.

1. Place the dates, pumpkin seeds, cocoa, 2 tablespoons of chocolate chips, and vanilla in the bowl of a food processor.

2. Pulse several times to break down the dates, then leave the processor on to blend until the mixture forms a ball, 30 to 45 seconds.

3. Transfer the large ball of "batter" to a piece of wax paper. Moisten your hands with water to prevent the batter from sticking, and divide it into 16 equal portions.

4. Roll each portion into a smooth ball. Dip the bottoms of each in the remaining 2 tablespoons of chocolate chips. Place the balls on a serving plate, chip-side up. Enjoy the bites right away, or chill them for 30 minutes or longer. The bites will firm up as they chill. Refrigerate in an airtight container for up to 4 days or freeze for up to 2 weeks.

SUBSTITUTION TIP *Use chopped nuts of your choice in place of the pumpkin seeds.*

PER SERVING (2 pieces): Calories: 184; Total fat: 2g; Total carbs: 42g; Sugar: 33g; Protein: 2g; Fiber: 4g; Sodium: 9mg

MAKES 8 (4-BY-1½-INCH) BARS

Prep time: 10 minutes, plus at least 1 hour to chill

COOK   ING

½ cup sunflower seed butter

2 tablespoons coconut oil

120 grams (about 1½ cups) purity protocol oats

½ cup toasted pumpkin seeds

⅓ cup sugar-free chocolate chips, plus 1 tablespoon for topping (optional)

Five-Ingredient No-Sugar Granola Bars

Egg-free • ***Vegetarian*** As someone with multiple food allergies, finding a great-tasting granola bar is no easy task. I created this recipe with no added sugar and a healthy dose of protein from sunflower seed butter. I use single-ingredient sunflower seed butter made with only toasted sunflower seeds. To keep these bars sugar-free, I use Lily's™ Dark Chocolate Premium Baking Chips, which have no added sugar.

1. Line the bottom and sides of an 8-by-8-inch pan with aluminum foil.

2. Place the sunflower seed butter and coconut oil in a large microwave-safe bowl. Microwave for 30 to 45 seconds, or just until softened. Stir.

3. Add the oats and pumpkin seeds and stir to coat. Stir in ⅓ cup of chocolate chips.

4. Spoon the mixture into the pan. Place a sheet of wax paper a few inches longer than the pan on top of the mixture and press down into an even layer. Remove the wax paper and sprinkle the remaining 1 tablespoon of chocolate chips on top (if using). Place the wax paper back over the mixture, then use the flat bottom of a drinking glass or measuring cup to press the mixture into the pan. Press firmly. This helps the bars stay together when you cut them.

5. Refrigerate for at least 1 hour. Lift the foil to remove the bars from the pan. Use a large, sharp knife to cut the granola into 8 rectangular bars. Refrigerate in an airtight container for up to 1 week.

VARIATION 1 **Peanut Butter Bars:** Substitute no-sugar-added peanut butter for the sunflower seed butter and chopped salted peanuts for the pumpkin seeds.

VARIATION 2 **Fruit and Seed Bars:** Omit the chocolate chips. Reduce the pumpkin seeds to ¼ cup and add ¼ cup of toasted sunflower seeds. Add ½ cup of dried fruit, such as tart cherries, blueberries, and/or raisins.

INGREDIENT TIP *If you do not have coconut oil, substitute ghee or butter. You may also add up to 1 tablespoon of honey (or pure maple syrup) for a sweeter bar.*

PER SERVING (1 bar): Calories: 197; Total fat: 16g; Total carbs: 11g; Sugar: 0g; Protein: 6g; Fiber: 1g; Sodium: 2mg

CHAPTER 6

Simple Sides

Side dishes are my favorite part of any meal. I can make a meal of just sides. If you think the only easy accompaniment to a meal is a plain salad, this chapter will change your mind. In the time you can get a green salad on the table, you can make most of these recipes.

Don't overlook the importance of putting thought into what you will serve with your main dish. Most of us focus on making the perfect roast, steak, or fish, but sides should not be an afterthought. What we serve alongside our main dish can make or break the meal.

Keeping variety on our plate also means we get a variety of nutrients in our diet. In the summertime, make the most of the farmers' market and buy local, fresh produce. You can use these recipes as guides and create some new dishes of your own.

7 medium carrots

Juice of ½ lime

2 tablespoons
sunflower oil

1 teaspoon
Dijon mustard

¼ teaspoon salt

⅛ teaspoon freshly
ground black pepper

1 teaspoon dried
cilantro or parsley

French Carrot Salad

Vegan Living in France, I learned that the secret to this classic French dish is how the carrots are grated. I use the smallest holes on a standard box grater. Do not buy pre-grated carrots for this dish. They are too coarse and will not be tender. There's no need to peel the carrots, though. Simply trim the ends as needed and use a vegetable brush to scrub them gently.

1. Trim off the ends of the carrots and gently scrub them under cool running water. Pat dry with paper towels.

2. Using the smallest holes on a box grater, grate the carrots into a shallow serving bowl.

3. In a small bowl, whisk together the lime juice, oil, mustard, salt, and pepper until smooth. Drizzle the dressing over the carrots, then sprinkle with the cilantro or parsley.

4. Very gently toss the carrots in the dressing and serve immediately.

VARIATION **Celery Root Salad:** Substitute half a large celery root for the carrots and prepare as directed.

INGREDIENT TIP *Organic sunflower oil or a similar neutral-tasting oil yields the most authentic flavor in this salad. Olive oil is too strongly flavored for this dish.*

PER SERVING Calories: 106; Total fat: 7g; Total carbs: 11g; Sugar: 5g; Protein: 1g; Fiber: 3g; Sodium: 235mg

SERVES 8

Prep time: 10 minutes

NO COOK | 5 ING | 30 MIN | 1 POT

Zest and juice of 1 lime

2 tablespoons extra-virgin olive oil

1 teaspoon salt

½ cup chopped fresh cilantro

1 medium avocado, diced

4 cups shredded purple cabbage

Cilantro-Lime Slaw

Vegan Forget what you know about white, gloppy, and soggy coleslaw. Think fresh, crisp, crunchy, and bright. There's a hint of creaminess from avocado here, and the lime juice brings a sweet citrus note that will complement every crisp-edged bit of barbecue you can imagine grilling. But the best place for this slaw? Right on top of Grilled Fish Tacos (page 151). You'll never eat them without it again!

1. In a large bowl, whisk together the lime zest and juice, oil, and salt.
2. Add the cilantro and avocado, and toss to coat.
3. Add the cabbage and toss gently to coat.
4. Serve immediately, or cover and refrigerate for up to 8 hours.

VARIATION 1 Creamy Mustard Slaw for Barbecue: Combine 2 tablespoons of yellow mustard, 2 tablespoons of mayonnaise, 1 tablespoon of sugar, 1 teaspoon of hot sauce, ½ teaspoon of salt, and ¼ teaspoon of black pepper in a large mixing bowl. Add 4 cups of shredded green cabbage and ½ cup of shredded carrot. Toss to coat. Refrigerate for at least 1 hour. Serve with Slow Cooker Barbecue Pork (page 178).

VARIATION 2 Pineapple-Jalapeño Slaw: To the original recipe dressing, add ½ cup of well-drained crushed pineapple and ½ tablespoon of minced jalapeño pepper. Toss with the cabbage and refrigerate for 1 hour before serving. This is excellent with grilled shrimp, shrimp tacos, or any Mexican dish.

PER SERVING Calories: 90; Total fat: 9g; Total carbs: 4g; Sugar: 1g; Protein: 1g; Fiber: 3g; Sodium: 299mg

Prep time: 5 minutes

Cook time: 10 minutes

ING   MIN   POT

1 medium
head cauliflower

1 cup Homemade
Chicken Stock (page 34)

½ teaspoon salt

4 garlic cloves, roasted,
or ½ teaspoon
garlic powder

2 tablespoons ghee or
dairy-free butter

Roasted Garlic Smashed Cauliflower

Dairy-free · *Egg-free* Even if you're not a cauliflower fan, don't turn away. This smashed cauliflower gives you the consistency of your favorite creamy mashed potatoes without the starch. It's great if you're avoiding nightshades, too. Pungent garlic turns sweet and creamy when roasted, so don't be shy about adding it. Ghee packs the most flavorful punch, but a dairy-free butter works great, too! To use a vegetable stock, refer to the substitution tip for Homemade Chicken Stock (page 34).

1. Cut out and discard the cauliflower core and any outer leaves or stems. Cut the cauliflower into florets and place them in a 2-quart or larger saucepan.

2. Place the saucepan over high heat and add the stock and salt. Cook, covered, for 5 minutes at a boil.

3. Uncover and cook 5 minutes more on high, or until the cauliflower is tender. Most of the stock will evaporate.

4. Remove from heat and add the garlic and ghee. Use an immersion blender to blend until completely smooth. Alternatively, transfer to a food processor, in batches if necessary, and process until smooth. (Note: Steam builds in the food processor with hot foods, so allow the cauliflower to cool a bit before processing.)

VARIATION 1 **Loaded Smashed Cauliflower Casserole:** Omit the salt, but otherwise prepare as directed. After blending smooth, spoon the mash into a serving dish and top with ½ cup of cooked, crumbled bacon, ½ cup of shredded Cheddar cheese, and 1 tablespoon of snipped fresh chives. Serve with a dollop of sour cream, if desired.

VARIATION 2 **Pesto Cauliflower Mash:** Prepare as directed. Stir in 2 tablespoons of pesto. Garnish with fresh basil.

INGREDIENT TIP *Anytime I roast vegetables, I add some garlic cloves to the pan to roast. Even if I don't use them right away, I cool and store them (unpeeled) in a jar in the refrigerator for up to 1 week. To use, simply open one end of the clove and squeeze out the roasted garlic as needed.*

PER SERVING Calories: 66; Total fat: 5g; Total carbs: 6g; Sugar: 2g; Protein: 2g; Fiber: 2g; Sodium: 350mg

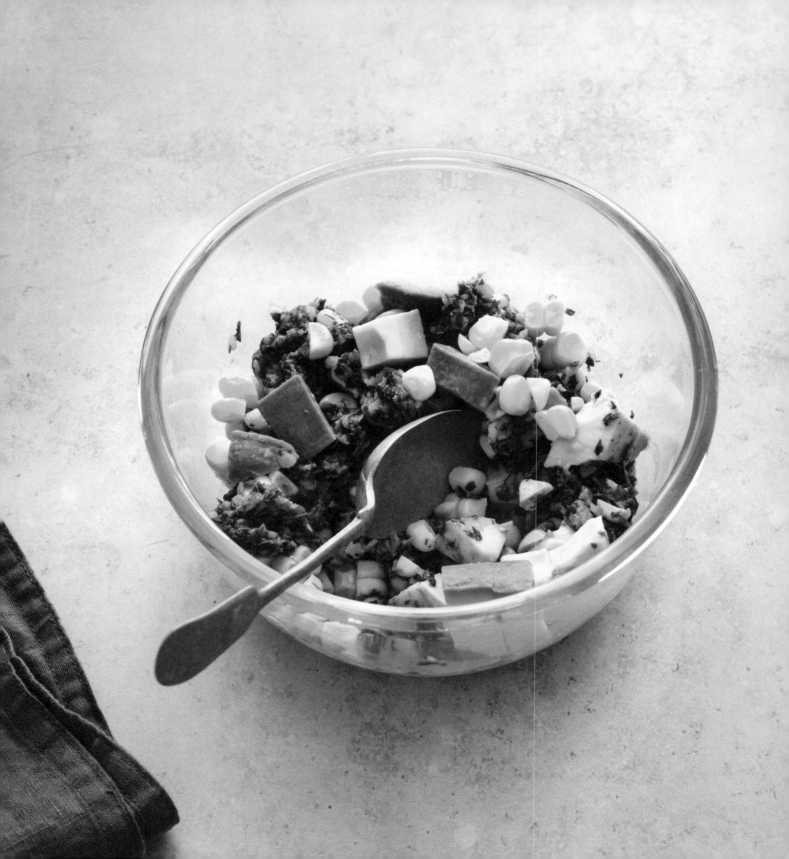

SERVES 4

Prep time: 10 minutes

NO COOK · 30 MIN

½ cup chopped fresh dill

½ cup chopped fresh cilantro

½ cup chopped fresh parsley

12 large basil leaves

¼ cup chopped sweet onion

1 tablespoon chopped jalapeño pepper

2 tablespoons extra-virgin olive oil

Juice of 1 lime

¼ teaspoon salt

1 ear fresh corn, kernels cut from the cob

1 avocado, diced

Corn-Avocado Salsa

Vegan This is a summertime staple at my house. Serve this no-cook salsa as an accompaniment to Grilled Fish Tacos (page 151) or any other seafood dish. It's also great with grilled poultry and meats or stirred into a bowl of shredded kale.

1. In the bowl of a food processor, combine the dill, cilantro, parsley, basil, onion, jalapeño, olive oil, lime juice, and salt. Pulse about 12 times, until blended but not smooth.

2. Transfer the mixture to a glass serving bowl and add the corn and avocado. Stir gently to incorporate. Cover and refrigerate until ready to serve.

VARIATION **Avocado-Only Salsa:** If you do not eat corn, omit it and use 2 avocados.

PER SERVING Calories: 204; Total fat: 17g; Total carbs: 13g; Sugar: 2g; Protein: 3g; Fiber: 5g; Sodium: 162mg

SERVES 6

Prep time: 10 minutes

Cook time: 30 minutes

¼ teaspoon coconut oil
or avocado oil

½ cup Quick Baking Mix
(page 26)

½ cup gluten-free
cornmeal

½ teaspoon salt

½ teaspoon
garlic powder

½ teaspoon
ground cumin

¼ teaspoon
cayenne pepper

1 (15-ounce) can
cream-style corn

1 (15-ounce) can whole
kernel corn, drained

2 large eggs

¼ cup diced roasted
red peppers

¼ cup fresh cilantro
leaves (optional)

2 tablespoons honey

2 tablespoons
dairy-free butter

Southern Corn Pudding

Dairy-free · ***Vegetarian*** If you're concerned about genetically modified organisms (GMOs), buy organic. In the United States, foods certified organic are also non-GMO foods. I use no-salt-added organic corn in this recipe; if you use salted corn, you may want to reduce or omit the salt called for in the ingredients. Also remember to buy certified gluten-free cornmeal to avoid cross-contamination issues.

1. Preheat the oven to 375°F. Grease a 2-quart baking dish with the oil.

2. In a large bowl, combine the baking mix, cornmeal, salt, garlic powder, cumin, and cayenne pepper, and whisk to blend.

3. Add the cream corn, corn kernels, eggs, roasted peppers, cilantro (if using), honey, and butter. Stir until no dry ingredients remain visible.

4. Spoon the mixture into the baking dish and bake for 30 minutes. Serve hot or warm.

VARIATION 1 **Spicy Corn Pudding:** Add ½ to 1 tablespoon of minced jalapeño pepper in step 3.

VARIATION 2 **Cheesy Corn Pudding:** Add 1 cup shredded sharp Cheddar cheese in step 3.

MAKE-AHEAD TIP *This recipe can be made a day ahead and stored, covered, in the refrigerator. Reheat in the oven until heated through, or microwave as desired.*

PER SERVING Calories: 225; Total fat: 7g; Total carbs: 39g; Sugar: 10g; Protein: 5g; Fiber: 3g; Sodium: 516mg

SERVES 4

Prep time: 5 minutes

Cook time: 10 minutes

1 tablespoon ghee

2 garlic cloves, minced

10 ounces baby
spinach leaves

½ cup heavy
(whipping) cream

¼ teaspoon
ground cardamom

¼ teaspoon freshly
ground black pepper

½ cup crumbled
goat cheese

Creamy Spinach with Cardamom

Egg-free · Vegetarian Pair this simple dish with grilled or baked fish, or serve it spooned over cooked rice for a comforting, meatless main or side. For the best results, use tender baby spinach leaves with all their stems removed.

1. Heat the ghee in a large skillet over medium heat. Add the garlic and sauté for 1 minute.

2. Add the spinach and stir until it wilts completely, about 4 minutes.

3. In a small bowl, whisk together the cream, cardamom, and pepper. Pour this into the skillet and add the cheese. Cook until heated through and serve.

VARIATION **Dairy-Free Creamy Spinach:** Use dairy-free butter instead of ghee, and substitute ½ cup of canned coconut cream for the heavy cream. Omit the cheese and add ¼ teaspoon of salt.

PER SERVING Calories: 160; Total fat: 15g; Total carbs: 4g; Sugar: 0g; Protein: 3g; Fiber: 2g; Sodium: 82mg

Prep time: 10 minutes

Cook time: 25 minutes

4 large russet potatoes

¼ cup avocado oil or coconut oil

½ teaspoon salt

½ teaspoon freshly ground black pepper

Crispy Oven Fries

Vegan Be sure to dry the potatoes well before cutting them into fries. I use avocado oil or coconut oil for high-heat cooking. Olive oil is not a good choice here because it doesn't hold up to higher temps.

1. Preheat the oven to 425°F. Line a large baking sheet or 2 smaller ones with parchment paper.

2. Scrub the potatoes well and dry completely with clean paper towels. If you prefer, you can peel the potatoes.

3. Cut the potatoes into ¼-inch-thick fries and place them in a large bowl. Pour the oil over the potatoes and toss to coat. Add the salt and pepper and toss again.

4. Place the fries on the baking sheet in a single layer, close to but not touching each other.

5. Bake for about 22 minutes, flipping the potatoes halfway through. The cooking time will vary depending on how thick or thin you cut your fries.

VARIATION **Garlic-Parmesan Fries:** When the fries are baked, transfer them to a large bowl and toss with 1 teaspoon of garlic powder and ½ cup of finely grated Parmesan cheese.

INGREDIENT TIP *Russet potatoes make fries with a crisp exterior and a tender, fluffy interior. If you use a different variety of potato, your results will vary.*

PER SERVING Calories: 373; Total fat: 14g; Total carbs: 58g; Sugar: 4g; Protein: 6g; Fiber: 9g; Sodium: 313mg

Prep time: 5 minutes

Cook time: 10 minutes

2 tablespoons
gluten-free soy sauce

1 tablespoon sesame oil

¼ teaspoon red
pepper flakes

½ tablespoon avocado
oil or coconut oil

2 cups riced cauliflower

½ cup sliced
water chestnuts

½ cup sliced mushrooms

½ cup julienned carrots

⅓ cup chopped
spring onions

1 garlic clove, minced

⅓ cup chopped
flat-leaf parsley

Fried Cauliflower Rice

Vegan If you're trying to cut carbs or just add more veggies to your plate, this dish is a great way to start. Serve it on its own or add cooked shrimp, diced cooked bacon, or leftover rotisserie chicken for a hearty, one-dish meal. You can also use a combination of cooked regular rice and cauliflower "rice" if you're not ready for a full-on cauliflower experience.

1. In a small bowl, whisk together the soy sauce, sesame oil, and red pepper flakes.

2. Heat the oil in a large skillet over high heat. Add the cauliflower, water chestnuts, mushrooms, carrots, and onions. Cook for 5 to 7 minutes, stirring often, until the vegetables start to become tender.

3. Add the garlic and cook for 1 minute more.

4. Remove the skillet from heat and add the sauce. Stir to coat the vegetables, then stir in the parsley and serve.

VARIATION **Caprese Cauliflower Rice:** Omit the soy sauce, sesame oil, red pepper flakes, water chestnuts, mushrooms, carrots, and parsley. Whisk together a dressing of 1 tablespoon of balsamic vinegar, 1 tablespoon of extra-virgin olive oil, and ⅛ teaspoon of salt. Add 1 cup of halved cherry tomatoes to the skillet with the cauliflower and onions. After removing the pan from heat, add the dressing and stir to coat. Stir in ½ cup of chopped basil leaves and ½ cup of cubed fresh mozzarella.

ALLERGEN TIP *For a soy-free dish, substitute coconut aminos for the gluten-free soy sauce.*

PER SERVING Calories: 154; Total fat: 11g; Total carbs: 13g; Sugar: 5g; Protein: 5g; Fiber: 5g; Sodium: 962mg

3 cups grated
sweet potatoes

2 large eggs

1 tablespoon
dried chives

½ teaspoon salt

½ teaspoon
baking powder

⅛ teaspoon freshly
ground black pepper

2 tablespoons
avocado oil or
coconut oil, divided

Sweet Potato Fritters

Dairy-free · ***Vegetarian*** With only a few ingredients, these crispy fritters are easy to put together quickly. For the best results, be sure your pan is very hot, but not smoking. Use an oil that is tolerant to high heat, like avocado oil or coconut oil. Serve these fritters with a side of bacon for breakfast, or as a side dish at dinner. White or orange sweet potatoes both work for this recipe.

1. In a large bowl, combine the sweet potatoes, eggs, chives, salt, baking powder, and black pepper and mix well.

2. Heat ½ tablespoon of oil at a time in a large skillet over high heat. Scoop ¼-cup portions of the sweet potato mixture into the skillet. Cook for about 2 minutes per side, then flip and cook for about 2 minutes more. Transfer to a plate. Repeat until all the mixture is used, adding more oil to the pan as needed. Serve the fritters hot.

VARIATION 1 **Hash Browns:** Substitute white potatoes for the sweet potatoes.

VARIATION 2 **Zucchini Fritters:** Substitute zucchini for the sweet potatoes.

PER SERVING Calories: 231; Total fat: 10g; Total carbs: 30g; Sugar: 10g; Protein: 6g; Fiber: 5g; Sodium: 380mg

SERVES 4

Prep time: 5 minutes

Cook time: 25 minutes

2 tablespoons coconut
oil or avocado oil, divided

1 head broccoli, cut into
bite-size florets

Zest of 1 lime

¼ teaspoon salt

Zesty Roasted Broccoli

Vegan If you're not a fan of steamed broccoli (or are simply bored by it), give roasting a try. This brings out an almost nutty flavor in the broccoli that you can't get with other preparation methods. If the kids need some extra motivation to eat their broccoli, serve it with a side of Ranch Dip (page 33). Leftovers are great to add to your next lunch salad.

1. Preheat the oven to 400°F. Line a baking sheet with aluminum foil and grease it with ¼ teaspoon of oil.

2. Place the broccoli florets on the prepared baking sheet in a single layer, then drizzle with the remaining oil and toss to coat.

3. Roast the broccoli for 12 minutes. Turn the florets, then roast for about 10 more minutes, until the broccoli is tender and turning brown and crisp at the edges.

4. Sprinkle with the lime zest and salt, toss to coat, and serve.

VARIATION 1 Zesty Roasted Cauliflower: Substitute cauliflower florets for the broccoli.

VARIATION 2 Saucy Asian Broccoli: Omit the lime zest and salt. While the broccoli roasts, whisk together 4 tablespoons of coconut aminos or gluten-free soy sauce, 2 tablespoons of sliced scallions, 1 tablespoon of rice vinegar, 2 teaspoons of sesame oil, and 1 teaspoon of minced ginger. Toss with the roasted broccoli before serving.

INGREDIENT TIP *Substitute lemon zest for the lime zest.*

PER SERVING Calories: 105; Total fat: 7g; Total carbs: 9g; Sugar: 2g; Protein: 4g; Fiber: 4g; Sodium: 192mg

CHAPTER 7

Dinner Salads

I started making what I call "bowl meals" years ago, before they were trendy. For me, this everything-in-one-bowl approach came from my meal prep days, when I cooked several different foods and wanted a taste of them all by the end of my cooking session. In fact, I believe the secret to great bowl meals is spending a few hours on the weekend prepping for the week ahead. I roast pans of sweet potatoes, white potatoes, carrots, and squash; I boil eggs, caramelize onions, and make a big batch of rice. I also make three sauces each week so I can add flavor to my dinner salads in a flash. Making a meal plan for the week is the key to success, and keeps your trip to the grocery store on track.

SERVES 2

Prep time: 25 minutes

Cook time: 5 minutes

1 cup cubed Cornbread
(page 189)

1 tablespoon Homemade
Ranch Seasoning
(page 33)

½ tablespoon
sunflower oil

1 cup cooked,
cubed chicken

¼ cup All-American
Barbecue Sauce
(page 32)

2 cups Cilantro-Lime
Slaw (page 73)

1 cup Fluffy Plain Rice
(see the first variation
on page 127)

½ cup Corn-Avocado
Salsa (page 77)

¼ cup thinly sliced
red onion

2 dill pickle spears,
sliced (optional)

Barbecue Chicken Salad Bowl

Dairy-free Make your work in the kitchen pull double duty. Most of the ingredients in this salad are recipes in the book, so you can make them ahead and use them for this dish and others, too. This recipe always makes my family's weekly menu plan when we have leftover Roasted Harissa Chicken (page 160).

1. In a medium bowl, toss the cornbread cubes with the ranch seasoning.

2. Heat the oil in a large skillet over medium-high heat. Add the cornbread and cook for 1 to 2 minutes per side, or until toasted. Remove the skillet from heat and set aside.

3. In a small saucepan over medium-low heat, toss the chicken with the barbecue sauce. Heat until warmed through. Alternatively, place in a microwave-safe bowl to heat.

4. Assemble the salads by dividing the chicken, slaw, rice, and salsa between 2 plates or bowls. Top each with the red onion, cornbread croutons, and pickle slices (if using).

VARIATION **Meatless Barbecue Bowl:** Omit the chicken. Substitute with roasted sweet potatoes tossed in the barbecue sauce.

INGREDIENT TIP *Store-bought gluten-free rotisserie chicken is a great option when time is short.*

PER SERVING Calories: 407; Total fat: 10g; Total carbs: 52g; Sugar: 4g; Protein: 26g; Fiber: 3g; Sodium: 380mg

SERVES 2

Prep time: 15 minutes

Cook time: 20 minutes

½ tablespoon coconut oil or avocado oil, divided

3 cups cubed butternut squash

6 strips bacon

1 tablespoon yellow mustard

3 cups shaved Brussels sprouts

¼ teaspoon salt

¼ teaspoon freshly ground black pepper

Brussels & Butternut Bowl with Crispy Bacon

Dairy-free • *Egg-free* No one in my family liked eating Brussels sprouts until I started to use shaved Brussels sprouts in meals. That was a game-changer. I simply pulse raw Brussels sprouts in the food processor until they have a sliced appearance. If you want a jump start on roasting the squash for this dish, microwave it for about 8 minutes, then cut the roasting time in half.

1. Preheat the oven to 400°F. Line a baking sheet with aluminum foil or grease it with ¼ teaspoon of oil.

2. Place the squash on the prepared baking sheet and drizzle it with the remaining oil. Toss to coat. Roast for 20 minutes, or until the squash is tender and beginning to brown on the edges.

3. While the squash roasts, cook the bacon. Place the bacon in a large, cold skillet over medium heat. Cook until crisp, turning it occasionally for even browning. Thinly sliced bacon will take 8 to 10 minutes, while thick-cut bacon will take 15 to 20 minutes. Transfer the bacon to a paper towel–lined plate to drain. Place 1 tablespoon of bacon grease in a small bowl and stir in the mustard. Leave the remaining bacon grease in the skillet.

4. Add the Brussels sprouts to the skillet. Cook over medium-high heat until tender and beginning to brown, about 8 minutes. Stir in the mustard mixture, then add the squash and toss to coat.

5. Season with the salt and pepper, and divide between 2 serving bowls. Crumble 3 slices of bacon over each bowl and serve.

VARIATION **Curry Sprout Salad with Chicken:** Omit the bacon and mustard. Whisk together 2 tablespoons of coconut milk and 1 teaspoon of curry powder to add to the sprouts after cooking. Plate the sprouts and squash, then top with sliced cooked chicken breast.

PER SERVING Calories: 455; Total fat: 28g; Total carbs: 28g; Sugar: 6g; Protein: 28g; Fiber: 8g; Sodium: 1726mg

Prep time: 15 minutes

Cook time: 15 minutes

30
MIN

FOR THE HONEY-MUSTARD SAUCE

2 tablespoons mayonnaise

1 tablespoon yellow mustard

½ tablespoon honey

⅛ teaspoon salt

⅛ teaspoon cayenne pepper

FOR THE BURGERS

8 ounces ground beef

¼ teaspoon garlic powder

¼ teaspoon onion powder

¼ teaspoon salt

2 slices Cheddar cheese or dairy-free Cheddar cheese

FOR THE SALAD

4 cups chopped romaine lettuce

1 medium tomato, seeded and diced

2 dill pickle spears

¼ cup sliced red onion

Cheeseburger Lovers' Salad

Dairy-free Burgers on buns are great, but I love a big cheeseburger salad sometimes. Change the cheese and seasonings for variety, add the toppings and condiments you love, and if you're looking for a full-on burger experience, add a side of Crispy Oven Fries (page 80).

1. Make the sauce by whisking together all of its ingredients in a small bowl. Set aside.

2. Make the burgers by putting the beef, garlic powder, onion powder, and salt in a medium bowl. With clean hands, mix the ingredients until well combined. Divide the mixture in half and form into 2 patties.

3. Place a large skillet over medium-high heat. Once the pan is hot, add the patties and cook for about 5 minutes per side for medium-done burgers, or until they reach your desired doneness. Turn off the heat, top each burger with a slice of cheese, and cover the pan to steam and melt the cheese, about 1 minute.

4. Make the salad by dividing the lettuce, tomato, pickles, and onion between 2 large plates. Top each with a burger and serve with the sauce.

VARIATION **Spicy Guac Burgers:** Substitute pepper jack cheese for the Cheddar. Omit the pickles and onion. Top the burgers with Ultimate Guacamole (page 58).

PER SERVING Calories: 562; Total fat: 43g; Total carbs: 18g; Sugar: 10g; Protein: 27g; Fiber: 3g; Sodium: 1625mg

SERVES 2

Prep time: 15 minutes

Cook time: 15 minutes

FOR THE CHIMICHURRI

½ cup flat-leaf
parsley, packed

3 fresh mint leaves

2 tablespoons
extra-virgin olive oil

1 tablespoon rice vinegar

1 garlic clove

¼ teaspoon salt

FOR THE SALAD

¼ teaspoon coconut
oil or avocado oil,
for greasing

2 (4-ounce) salmon fillets

8 asparagus spears

1 cup Coconut Rice (see
the second variation on
page 127)

½ cup shredded carrots

4 radishes, thinly sliced

Chimichurri Salmon Salad

Dairy-free · Egg-free Chimichurri is a condiment that originated in Argentina. It's traditionally served with beef or chicken, but it adds new life to baked salmon. It's typically stirred together, not pulsed in the food processor, but I like the shortcut for chopping the parsley. Don't worry about plucking individual leaves from the parsley; soft stems are fine in chimichurri.

TO MAKE THE CHIMICHURRI

Place all the ingredients in the bowl of a food processor. Pulse several times to roughly chop.

TO MAKE THE SALAD

1. Preheat the oven to 375°F. Line a baking sheet with aluminum foil or grease lightly with the oil.

2. Place the salmon and asparagus on the prepared baking sheet. Spread half the chimichurri across the top of the fillets. Bake for 15 minutes.

3. While the salmon bakes, divide the rice, carrots, and radishes between 2 serving plates. Top the rice with the salmon. Serve with the asparagus and remaining chimichurri.

VARIATION 1 **Cilantro Chimichurri:** Substitute fresh cilantro for the parsley. Omit the mint.

VARIATION 2 **Paleo Bowl:** Substitute Fried Cauliflower Rice (page 81) for the coconut rice.

PER SERVING Calories: 552; Total fat: 29g; Total carbs: 35g; Sugar: 4g; Protein: 32g; Fiber: 4g; Sodium: 411mg

SERVES 2

Prep time: 15 minutes

Cook time: 20 minutes

FOR THE SALAD

2 (3-inch) ears fresh corn

4 strips bacon

2 hard-boiled eggs

4 cups baby
spinach leaves

6 ounces cooked
chicken, cubed

1 avocado, diced

1 medium tomato, diced

¼ cup crumbled
goat cheese (optional)

Chives, for garnish
(optional)

FOR THE VINAIGRETTE

1 cup fresh or
frozen strawberries

3 tablespoons
extra-virgin olive oil

½ tablespoon
balsamic vinegar

¼ teaspoon salt

⅛ teaspoon freshly
ground black pepper

Cobb Salad with Strawberry Vinaigrette

Dairy-free Why prepare corn, bacon, and eggs just for this meal? To get a jump start on future meals, cook extra of all three! Use the bacon in a Brussels & Butternut Bowl (page 87), cut off corn kernels and use them in Corn-Avocado Salsa (page 77), and make a batch of Traditional Deviled Eggs (page 62) for a snack or side. There's extra vinaigrette for a future meal, too.

1. Place the corn in a medium saucepan and add just enough water to cover. Turn the heat to high and boil for 6 minutes. Remove from heat, drain the water, and cover the pan until ready to serve.

2. While the corn cooks in the saucepan, place the bacon in a large skillet over medium-high heat. Cook, flipping as needed, until crisp, about 5 minutes. Transfer the bacon to a paper towel–lined plate to drain.

3. Peel and slice the eggs.

4. Divide the spinach, chicken, avocado, tomato, and cheese (if using) between 2 salad bowls. Top each with crumbled bacon and egg slices.

5. Make the vinaigrette by putting all of its ingredients in the bowl of a food processor. Blend until smooth.

6. Drizzle 2 tablespoons of dressing over each salad. Sprinkle with chives (if using), and serve with the corn on the side. You can refrigerate leftover vinaigrette in an airtight container for up to 4 days.

VARIATION Club Cobb: Substitute turkey for the chicken. Substitute shredded iceberg lettuce for the spinach. Omit the corn, use shredded Cheddar cheese instead of goat cheese, and add dill pickle slices. For the dressing: Whisk together 2 tablespoons of apple cider vinegar, 2 tablespoons of extra-virgin olive oil, 1 teaspoon of minced garlic, and 1 teaspoon of Dijon mustard. Season to taste with salt and pepper.

MAKE-AHEAD TIP *Use leftover Roasted Harissa Chicken (page 160) to save time.*

PER SERVING Calories: 936; Total fat: 64g; Total carbs: 35g; Sugar: 9g; Protein: 63g; Fiber: 12g; Sodium: 1331mg

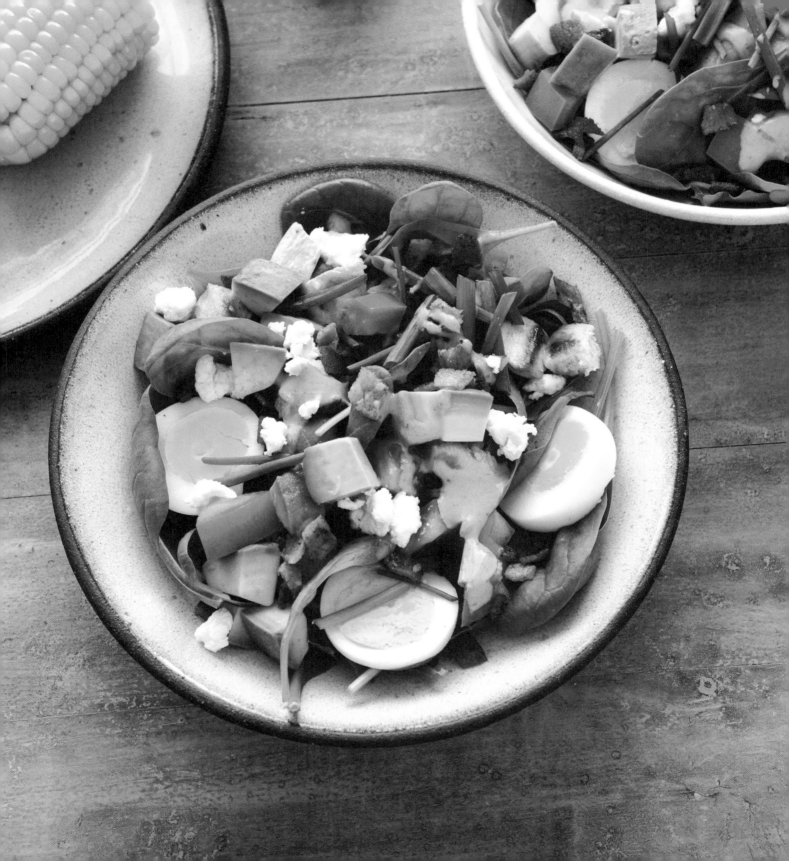

SERVES 2

Prep time: 15 minutes

Cook time: 25 minutes

1½ tablespoons coconut oil, melted, divided

1 cup diced sweet potato

1 tablespoon flaxseed meal

1 tablespoon freshly squeezed lemon juice

1 garlic clove, minced

½ teaspoon salt, divided

3 cups chopped kale

2 (4-ounce) salmon fillets

¼ teaspoon freshly ground black pepper

1 cup Zesty Roasted Broccoli (page 83)

1 avocado, diced

½ cup fresh blueberries

Superfood Salad

Dairy-free · Egg-free This salad packs a powerful nutritional punch. Colorful, energy-filled, and flavorful foods like these are the perfect example of how a naturally gluten-free diet can work for you. Get the most nutrients out of fruits and vegetables by using what's in season. They naturally taste better, too!

1. Preheat the oven to 425°F. Grease a baking sheet with ½ tablespoon of the oil.

2. Place the diced sweet potato on the prepared baking sheet and stir to coat with the oil on the sheet. Roast until tender, about 10 minutes.

3. While the sweet potato chunks roast, make the salad dressing. In a large bowl, put the remaining tablespoon of coconut oil, the flaxseed meal, lemon juice, garlic, and ¼ teaspoon of salt. Whisk to combine. Add the kale. Using your fingers, massage the dressing into the kale for tender greens.

4. Divide the kale between 2 serving bowls and top with the sweet potato.

5. Reduce the oven temperature to 375°F. Place the salmon on the baking sheet and season it with the remaining ¼ teaspoon of salt and the pepper. Bake for about 15 minutes, or until desired doneness.

6. Top each bowl of greens and sweet potato with the salmon, broccoli, avocado, and blueberries. Serve immediately.

VARIATION **Superfood Salad 2:** Substitute butternut squash for the sweet potato, beet greens for the kale, asparagus for the broccoli, and strawberries for the blueberries.

ALLERGEN TIP *If you do not eat coconut oil, use avocado oil instead. For flaxseed meal, substitute chia seeds.*

PER SERVING Calories: 642; Total fat: 38g; Total carbs: 50g; Sugar: 12g; Protein: 31g; Fiber: 15g; Sodium: 735mg

Prep time: 15 minutes

Cook time: 20 minutes

1 pound new potatoes

1 tablespoon coconut oil or avocado oil

4 large eggs

8 slices bacon

¼ cup extra-virgin olive oil

2 tablespoons rice vinegar

1 tablespoon whole-grain mustard

¼ cup chopped flat-leaf parsley

2 tablespoons chopped fresh dill

2 tablespoons chopped fresh chives

½ teaspoon salt

⅛ teaspoon freshly ground black pepper

1 small red onion, halved and thinly sliced

¼ cup pitted green olives, chopped

¼ cup pickle slices

Deconstructed Potato Salad Bowl

Dairy-free Skip the mayo-laden version of potato salad for this lighter, deconstructed dish. This is perfect as a side dish at your next backyard barbecue, but also makes a great dinner salad because it's very filling.

1. Preheat the oven to 425°F.

2. Scrub and dry the potatoes. Cut them in half and place in a medium bowl. Add the oil and toss to coat. Arrange in a single layer on a baking sheet. Roast until tender and brown around the edges, about 20 minutes.

3. While the potatoes roast, place the eggs in a saucepan and cover with water. Place over high heat and boil for 6 minutes. Drain off the water and refill the pan with ice and water to quickly chill the eggs. Once cool, drain the water and peel the eggs.

4. While the potatoes roast and the eggs cook, place a large skillet over medium-high heat. Add the bacon and fry, turning as needed, until crisp, about 5 minutes. Transfer to a paper towel–lined plate to drain.

5. In a large serving bowl, whisk together the olive oil, vinegar, and mustard. Add the parsley, dill, chives, salt, and pepper and whisk to combine. Add the roasted potatoes to the bowl and toss with the dressing.

6. Halve the eggs and place them around the inside edge of the bowl. Add the onion, olives, and pickle slices on top of the potatoes. Crumble the bacon on top. Serve at room temperature.

VARIATION 1 **Cauliflower Salad:** If you're watching your carb intake, substitute cauliflower for the potatoes.

VARIATION 2 **Sweet Potato Salad:** Substitute cubed sweet potatoes for the new potatoes. Omit the eggs, olives, and pickles. Add ½ cup of crumbled goat cheese, ¼ cup of dried cranberries, and ¼ cup of toasted pumpkin seeds.

PER SERVING Calories: 549; Total fat: 40g; Total carbs: 24g; Sugar: 3g; Protein: 24g; Fiber: 4g; Sodium: 1748mg

1 tablespoon
coconut oil, plus
¼ teaspoon (optional)

1 large ripe plantain

¼ teaspoon salt

¼ teaspoon freshly
ground black pepper

2 cups chopped kale

1 cup Mexican Rice
(page 126)

1 cup canned black
beans, drained
and rinsed

½ cup cucumber slices

¼ cup salsa

Latin Dinner Salad

Vegan One of my favorite restaurants serves delicious Latin-American food. This is my take on their vegetable plate dinner. I serve it in a large salad bowl with a drizzle of spicy sriracha.

1. Preheat the oven to 425°F and line a baking sheet with aluminum foil or grease it with ¼ teaspoon of oil.

2. Peel the plantain and slice it into ½-inch-thick slices.

3. In a medium bowl, combine the plantain slices, 1 tablespoon of coconut oil, the salt, and pepper. Toss to coat. Place the plantains in a single layer on the prepared baking sheet. Roast for about 10 minutes, until tender and beginning to brown.

4. Divide the kale, rice, and beans between 2 large salad bowls. Place the plantains over the kale. Serve with the cucumber and salsa.

VARIATION **Meat Lovers' Latin Bowl:** Add ½ cup of chopped cooked chicken or steak to each bowl.

SUBSTITUTION TIP *If you don't like kale, use another dark, leafy green, like spinach.*

PER SERVING Calories: 448; Total fat: 8g; Total carbs: 85g; Sugar: 15g; Protein: 15g; Fiber: 12g; Sodium: 621mg

1 tablespoon
sunflower oil

3 cups cubed Cornbread
(page 189)

¼ cup extra-virgin
olive oil

2 teaspoons rice vinegar

1 garlic clove, minced

2 cups cubed
tomatoes, drained

½ teaspoon salt

¼ teaspoon freshly
ground black pepper

½ cup baby
spinach leaves

Southern-Style Panzanella

Dairy-free* • *Vegetarian Every time I make Cornbread (page 189), I use the leftovers to make this dish. It's my Southern twist on classic Italian tomato-bread salad. Sometimes I serve it with a bowl of crumbled goat cheese or feta at the table to satisfy the cheese lovers.

1. Heat the oil in a large skillet over medium-high heat. Add the cornbread cubes and toast until golden all over, about 10 minutes.

2. In a small bowl, whisk together the olive oil, vinegar, and garlic.

3. In a large serving bowl, toss the tomatoes with the salt and pepper. Add the cornbread croutons and toss again. Drizzle the vinaigrette over the salad and toss until the dressing is absorbed by the croutons.

4. Just before serving, add the spinach leaves and toss together.

VARIATION 1 **Traditional Panzanella:** Use leftover Top 8–Free Sandwich Bread (page 191) instead of the cornbread and omit the spinach.

VARIATION 2 **Caprese Panzanella:** Add ½ cup of torn basil leaves and 1 cup of cubed fresh mozzarella to the traditional variation above.

MAKE-AHEAD TIP *Make the cornbread during your meal prep day. Cube the cornbread in advance. It will dry out just enough to crisp to perfection when toasted.*

PER SERVING Calories: 192; Total fat: 13g; Total carbs: 17g; Sugar: 2g; Protein: 3g; Fiber: 1g; Sodium: 413mg

CHAPTER 8

Soups & Stews

Soup and stews are forgiving and adaptable. If they turn out too thick, add more liquid. Water always works, or add more of whatever liquid is used in the recipe. For a soup that's too thin, add a mixture of cornstarch and cold water (called a slurry) to boiling soup. Start with 1 tablespoon of cornstarch to 2 tablespoons of cold water. Stir into the soup and give it a few minutes to thicken. Adding a small amount of instant potato flakes or a puréed vegetable like cauliflower, potato, or sweet potato are also excellent ways to thicken soup or stew.

Soups and stews always taste even better on the second day. Flavors have time to meld after a night in the refrigerator. Most soups keep well in the refrigerator for three or four days and will freeze well for up to a month.

Prep time: 15 minutes

Pressure cooking time:
50 minutes

POT

2 pounds boneless leg of
lamb, cut into chunks

1 large white potato,
peeled and cubed

1 large sweet potato,
peeled and cubed

1 rutabaga, peeled
and cubed

2 large carrots, sliced

2 parsnips, sliced

1 medium onion, diced

3 rosemary sprigs

1½ teaspoons salt

1½ teaspoons
garlic powder

1 teaspoon ground sage

⅛ teaspoon freshly
ground black pepper

2 tablespoons Gigi's
Everyday Gluten-Free
Flour (page 27)

2 cups water

Pressure Cooker Lamb Stew

Dairy-free · Egg-free Make a pass through the produce aisle, and you'll have most of the ingredients for this hearty stew. Ask the butcher to cube the lamb for you, or do what I do—buy a leg of lamb, cube it yourself, and then save the rest for another recipe. It's a huge money-saver. This is a forgiving recipe. If you don't like a vegetable in it, swap it out for an equal amount of something you do like.

1. In your pressure cooker pot, place the lamb, white potato, sweet potato, rutabaga, carrots, parsnips, onion, rosemary, salt, garlic powder, sage, and pepper.

2. In a small bowl, whisk the flour into the water. Pour this into the pressure cooker.

3. Lock the lid into place. Cook at high pressure for 50 minutes. After cooking, naturally release the pressure for 15 minutes, then quick release any remaining pressure. Unlock and remove the lid.

4. Remove and discard the rosemary sprigs. Stir and serve.

VARIATION **Slow Cooker Lamb Stew:** Follow steps 1 and 2 in the recipe, placing the ingredients in a 6-quart slow cooker. Cover and cook on low for 8 hours. Remove the rosemary sprigs and serve.

INGREDIENT TIP *If you can't find lamb, or if lamb isn't in your budget, substitute an equal amount of cubed beef stew meat.*

PER SERVING Calories: 438; Total fat: 14g; Total carbs: 37g; Sugar: 10g; Protein: 38g; Fiber: 7g; Sodium: 613mg

Prep time: 5 minutes

Pressure cooking time:
15 minutes

30 MIN **1** POT

1 (14-ounce) can
light coconut milk

1¾ cups water

1 cup red lentils, rinsed

1 cup grated
sweet potato

½ cup diced onion

1 teaspoon garlic powder

1 teaspoon salt

⅛ teaspoon
cayenne pepper

Pressure Cooker Red Lentil Soup

Vegan This simple soup is flavorful and comforting. Serve it on its own or ladle it over rice for a heartier meal. I specify using light coconut milk because full-fat is too heavy for this dish. Bear in mind that the soup thickens considerably as it cools. After refrigeration, add liquid when reheating to thin the consistency to your liking.

1. Place all the ingredients in the pressure cooker pot and stir.

2. Lock the lid into place. Cook at high pressure for 15 minutes. After cooking, naturally release the pressure. Unlock and remove the lid.

3. Stir and serve.

VARIATION 1 **Stove-top Red Lentil Soup:** Sauté the sweet potato and onion in ½ tablespoon of coconut oil over high heat until tender, about 5 minutes. Add the remaining ingredients, bring to a boil, then cover and reduce the heat to low. Simmer for 20 minutes, or until the lentils are tender.

VARIATION 2 **Lentil Vegetable Soup:** Omit the sweet potato. Add ½ cup of grated carrot and ½ cup of diced celery. Use 1¾ cups of vegetable stock instead of water. Stir in 1 tablespoon of freshly squeezed lemon juice and 2 tablespoons of chopped fresh parsley prior to serving.

INGREDIENT TIP *Red lentils are the fastest-cooking legumes, because the husks are removed and they are already split. Substituting other types of lentils in this recipe will not work with the specified cooking time.*

PER SERVING Calories: 186; Total fat: 4g; Total carbs: 30g; Sugar: 3g; Protein: 10g; Fiber: 11g; Sodium: 419mg

Prep time: 5 minutes

Cook time: 8 hours

POT

1 (15-ounce) can tomatoes, whole or diced, undrained

1 (14-ounce) can salt-free green beans, undrained

1 cup Homemade Vegetable Stock (see substitution tip on page 34)

2 medium russet potatoes, peeled and cubed

1 large sweet potato, peeled and cubed

1 medium onion, diced

1 cup corn kernels, fresh or frozen

3 tablespoons tomato paste

1 teaspoon dried dill

1 teaspoon salt

½ teaspoon garlic powder

½ teaspoon ground turmeric

⅛ teaspoon freshly ground black pepper (optional)

Slow Cooker Garden Vegetable Soup

Vegan This is my go-to vegetable soup recipe. It's easy to make year-round, and during the summer, I use fresh produce from my local farmers' market. When that's not available, I rely on organic frozen and canned veggies. Feel free to switch up the herbs and seasonings to suit your tastes.

1. Place all the ingredients in a 6-quart slow cooker. Cover and cook on low for 8 hours.

2. Refrigerate leftovers in an airtight container for up to 3 days. For longer storage, portion the soup into individual airtight serving containers and freeze for up to 1 month.

VARIATION **Pressure Cooker Garden Vegetable Soup:** Place the ingredients in your pressure cooker, lock the lid into place, and cook at high pressure for 35 minutes. Naturally release the pressure for at least 10 minutes, then quick release any remaining pressure.

SUBSTITUTION TIP *Substitute vegetables as you like. For example, swap out the potatoes and sweet potato for other root vegetables like carrots, parsnips, or turnips. Use sliced leeks instead of the onion. If you prefer, omit the corn. Use your imagination and let your preferences guide you.*

PER SERVING Calories: 81; Total fat: 0g; Total carbs: 18g; Sugar: 5g; Protein: 3g; Fiber: 4g; Sodium: 291mg

SERVES 2

Prep time: 5 minutes

NO COOK · 5 ING · 30 MIN · 1 POT

1 cup unsweetened coconut milk

1 medium cucumber, quartered

½ cup packed fresh cilantro or flat-leaf parsley

½ avocado, halved, pitted, and peeled

5 fresh mint leaves

¼ teaspoon salt

Creamy Chilled Green Soup

Vegan Cold soup never appealed to me until I had a version of this one in Paris a few years ago. It was served in a tall glass with a straw as a to-go healthy lunch option. It was so refreshing, filling, and flavorful that I had to recreate it at home. Leave the peel on the cucumber and use the cilantro stems. They are both full of flavor and nutrients.

1. Place all the ingredients in the bowl of a food processor or blender and blend until smooth.

2. Divide the soup between two glasses or bowls and serve immediately.

VARIATION **Spicy Chilled Soup:** Add fresh jalapeño pepper to taste and a squeeze of lime juice.

INGREDIENT TIP *Avocado makes this a creamy soup. If you prefer a thinner version, omit it.*

ALLERGEN TIP *If you cannot eat coconut, substitute the coconut milk with your favorite dairy-free milk.*

PER SERVING Calories: 301; Total fat: 29g; Total carbs: 13g; Sugar: 7g; Protein: 4g; Fiber: 4g; Sodium: 313mg

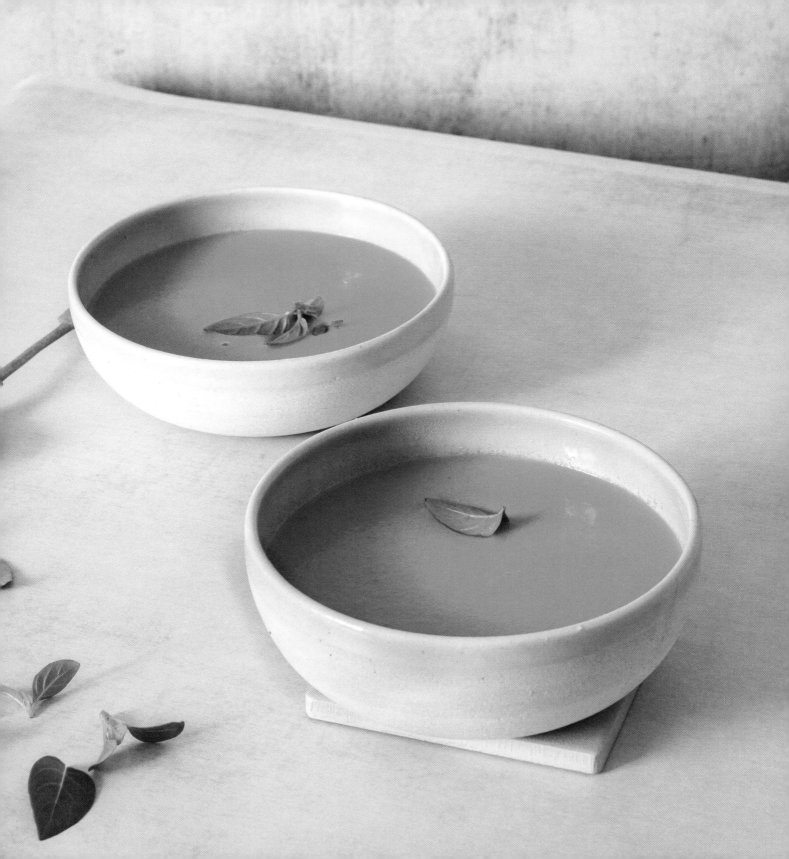

SERVES 4

Prep time: 5 minutes

Cook time: 15 minutes

5 ING · 30 MIN · 1 POT

1 (28-ounce) can whole or diced tomatoes, undrained

¾ cup unsweetened coconut milk

½ teaspoon salt

¼ teaspoon onion powder

⅛ teaspoon freshly ground black pepper

5 fresh basil leaves (optional)

Extra-virgin olive oil (optional)

Creamy Tomato Soup

Vegan This is a rare case in which canned is better than fresh. Whole or diced canned tomatoes give soups a richer tomato flavor. The coconut milk I use is from a carton, however, not a can. Try this soup with Salted Fennel Crackers (page 184) for a classic combo!

1. Place all the ingredients in a medium saucepan over medium heat.

2. Using an immersion blender, purée into a soup. Alternatively, place the ingredients in a blender, in batches if necessary, and blend until smooth, then transfer to the saucepan to heat.

3. Warm the soup for about 15 minutes, stirring occasionally. To serve, garnish with fresh basil and a drizzle of olive oil (if using).

VARIATION **Tomato Soup with Pasta and Parm:** Add 2 cups of cooked gluten-free pasta to the soup after blending. Top each serving with 1 tablespoon of grated Parmesan cheese.

INGREDIENT TIP *You can use any dairy or dairy-free milk in place of the coconut milk.*

PER SERVING Calories: 140; Total fat: 11g; Total carbs: 10g; Sugar: 6g; Protein: 3g; Fiber: 3g; Sodium: 307mg

Prep time: 5 minutes

Cook time: 15 minutes

1 tablespoon
dairy-free butter

3½ cups mixed
sliced mushrooms

2 cups unsweetened
coconut milk

1 cup Homemade
Vegetable Stock (see
substitution tip on
page 34)

¼ cup Gigi's Everyday
Gluten-Free Flour
(page 27)

½ teaspoon
garlic powder

½ teaspoon
onion powder

½ teaspoon salt

⅛ teaspoon freshly
ground black pepper

Creamy Dairy-Free Mushroom Soup

Vegan For the best flavor, use a variety of mushrooms in this recipe. I prefer a mixture of white, cremini, baby portobello, and shiitake mushrooms. You can enjoy this soup on its own or use it as an ingredient anywhere you need mushroom soup.

1. In a large saucepan, melt the butter over medium heat. Add the mushrooms and cook until they are tender, about 5 minutes.

2. Add the coconut milk, stock, flour, garlic powder, onion powder, salt, and pepper. Whisk vigorously to incorporate the flour into the liquids. Cook, stirring occasionally, until the mixture comes to a boil. Turn off the heat and let the soup sit for about 5 minutes. It will thicken as it cools.

SUBSTITUTION TIP *If you don't eat coconut, you can use any other dairy-free milk in place of the coconut milk. If you eat dairy products, you can use dairy butter and milk.*

PER SERVING Calories: 349; Total fat: 32g; Total carbs: 14g; Sugar: 6g; Protein: 6g; Fiber: 4g; Sodium: 542mg

SERVES 6

Prep time: 15 minutes, plus overnight to soak

Pressure cooking time: 35 minutes

1 pound dried
black beans

½ cup diced onion

½ cup diced celery

½ cup diced tomato

¼ cup chopped
green olives

4 garlic cloves, minced

2 teaspoons finely
diced jalapeño pepper

1½ teaspoons
ground cumin

1½ teaspoons salt

½ teaspoon
dried oregano

Juice of ½ lime

4 cups water

Pressure Cooker Cuban Black Bean Soup

Vegan The combination of vegetables, olives, jalapeños, and spices makes this soup very flavorful. To take the flavor to the next level, you can substitute Homemade Chicken Stock or the beef variation (page 34) for all, or part, of the water.

1. Rinse and drain the beans. Place them in a large bowl and cover with cold water by 2 inches. Refrigerate overnight to soak.

2. Drain the beans. Place them in the pressure cooker pot and add all of the remaining ingredients.

3. Lock the lid into place. Cook at high pressure for 35 minutes. After cooking, let the pressure release naturally. Unlock and remove the lid.

4. Using an immersion blender, purée some of the beans for added creaminess. Alternatively, transfer 2 cups of cooled soup to a blender and pulse about 10 times. Stir it back into the soup before serving.

5. Serve the soup as is, or with toppings such as guacamole, sour cream, diced hard-boiled egg, crisp bacon crumbles, diced ham, jalapeño slices, and shredded cheese.

VARIATION 1 **Slow Cooker Black Bean Soup:** Place the soaked, drained beans and remaining ingredients in a 6-quart slow cooker. Cover and cook on high for 8 hours.

VARIATION 2 **Black Bean Soup with Ham:** Add 1 to 2 cups diced cooked ham to the soup with the other ingredients.

PER SERVING Calories: 287; Total fat: 3g; Total carbs: 51g; Sugar: 3g; Protein: 17g; Fiber: 13g; Sodium: 774mg

POT

2 pounds grass-fed
ground beef

1 (28-ounce) can
whole tomatoes

3 cups riced cauliflower
or 1 (12-ounce) bag
frozen riced cauliflower

1 (6-ounce) can
tomato paste

1 cup diced onion

¼ cup salsa verde

3 garlic cloves, minced

1 tablespoon
chili powder

1 teaspoon
ground cumin

½ teaspoon salt

Easy Pressure Cooker Chili

Dairy-free · Egg-free This chili is the perfect base for toppings. Depending on your dietary preferences, choose from Ultimate Guacamole (page 58), shredded cheese, minced red onion, or sour cream. You could even crumble one of the Corn Muffins with Jalapeño and Cheddar (see the variation on page 189) on top. If you're not in a hurry, try the slow cooker variation below.

1. Place all the ingredients in the pressure cooker pot and stir to combine.

2. Lock the lid into place. Cook at high pressure for 35 minutes. After cooking, let the pressure release naturally for 15 minutes, then quick release any remaining pressure. Unlock and remove the lid.

3. Stir the chili and serve.

VARIATION 1 **Paleo Turkey Chili:** Substitute ground turkey for the beef.

VARIATION 2 **Chili with Beans:** Reduce the meat to 1 pound and add 2 (15-ounce) cans of drained black beans or kidney beans.

MAKE-AHEAD TIP *Place all the ingredients in a 6-quart slow cooker. Cover and cook on low for 8 hours.*

PER SERVING Calories: 237; Total fat: 12g; Total carbs: 17g; Sugar: 9g; Protein: 18g; Fiber: 5g; Sodium: 365mg

Prep time: 5 minutes

Pressure cooking time:
25 minutes

ING MIN POT

4 cups fresh or frozen
cauliflower florets

2 cups Homemade
Vegetable Stock (see
substitution tip on
page 34)

1 (14-ounce) can light
coconut milk

1 cup vegan pepper jack
cheese shreds

½ teaspoon salt

⅛ teaspoon freshly
ground black pepper

Pressure Cooker Spicy Cream of Cauliflower Soup

Vegan Some of my favorite foods are cauliflower, broccoli, cabbage, and Brussels sprouts—all members of the Brassica family of vegetables. My family doesn't share my enthusiasm, so I've had to create exceptional recipes to win them over. This soup is one that changed opinions about cauliflower in my house.

1. Place all the ingredients in the pressure cooker pot and stir to combine.

2. Lock the lid into place. Cook at high pressure for 25 minutes. After cooking, let the pressure release naturally. Unlock and remove the lid.

3. Using an immersion blender, blend the soup until smooth. Alternatively, allow the soup to cool, then transfer it, in batches if necessary, to a blender to purée until smooth. If the soup is blended while too hot, steam will build up and can blow the top of the blender right off.

VARIATION 1 **Stove-top Cauliflower Soup:** Place all the ingredients in a large soup pot and bring to a boil over high heat. Reduce the heat to low and cover the pot. Simmer for 45 minutes, or until the cauliflower is very tender. Purée with an immersion blender.

VARIATION 2 **Non-Vegan Cauliflower Soup:** Substitute Homemade Chicken Stock (page 34) for the vegetable stock; use regular milk and cheese.

PER SERVING Calories: 121; Total fat: 10g; Total carbs: 6g; Sugar: 2g; Protein: 2g; Fiber: 2g; Sodium: 509mg

Prep time: 15 minutes

Cook time: 1 hour
10 minutes

4 (1-inch-thick) slices
Top 8–Free Sandwich
Bread (page 191)

4 cups sliced
yellow onions

¼ cup ghee

½ teaspoon salt, plus
more for seasoning

1 quart low-sodium
beef stock

2 bay leaves

⅛ teaspoon freshly
ground black pepper

1½ cups grated
Comté cheese

French Onion Soup

Egg-free This soup takes some time to cook, but it is easy to make. If you don't have homemade stock handy, use a low-sodium store-bought stock. Just make sure it's gluten-free. The secrets to success with this soup are properly caramelizing the onions and using toasted Top 8–Free Sandwich Bread (page 191) and Comté cheese.

1. Preheat the oven to 375°F. Line a baking sheet with aluminum foil.

2. Place the bread slices on the baking sheet and toast on each side for about 10 minutes, or until the bread is dry and very crisp. Set aside. Increase the oven temperature to 400°F.

3. Place the onions, ghee, and salt in a large stockpot. Cook over medium-high heat to melt the ghee and get the pot sizzling, then reduce the heat to low. Cover and cook, stirring occasionally, until the onions are very soft and deep brown, 30 to 40 minutes.

4. Add the stock and bay leaves to the pot. Increase the heat to medium-high and bring to a boil. Boil for 10 minutes, then turn off the heat. Remove and discard the bay leaves. Season to taste with additional salt and the pepper.

5. Ladle the soup into 4 oven-safe soup crocks. Place the crocks on a large sheet pan. Top each crock with a slice of toasted bread, then divide the cheese evenly on top of the toasts.

6. Carefully transfer the sheet pan with the crocks to the oven. Bake for 15 to 20 minutes, until the cheese is melted and beginning to brown on top. Serve immediately. Note: The bowls will be very hot.

VARIATION **Vegetarian Onion Soup:** Substitute vegetable stock for the beef stock.

SUBSTITUTION TIP *Use Emmenthaler or Gruyère instead of the Comté cheese, and/or use butter instead of the ghee.*

PER SERVING Calories: 278; Total fat: 17g; Total carbs: 20g; Sugar: 6g; Protein: 12g; Fiber: 3g; Sodium: 669mg

Prep time: 10 minutes

Cook time: 8 hours

POT

1 (16-ounce) bag frozen black-eyed peas

1 (16-ounce) bag frozen chopped collard greens

1 small yellow onion, chopped

¾ cup water or Homemade Vegetable Stock (see substitution tip on page 34)

¼ cup apple cider vinegar

2 garlic cloves, minced

1 tablespoon dairy-free butter

½ teaspoon red pepper flakes

½ teaspoon salt

⅛ teaspoon freshly ground black pepper

Slow Cooker Luck & Money

Vegan Luck & Money is a twist on the classic Southern New Year's Day meal of black-eyed peas and collard greens. Serve this soup with Corn Muffins with Jalapeño and Cheddar (see the variation on page 189) and a glass of champagne. Cheers to the New Year!

Place all the ingredients in a 6-quart slow cooker. Cover and cook on low for 8 hours.

VARIATION 1 **Pressure Cooker Luck & Money:** Place all the ingredients in the pressure cooker pot. Cook at high pressure for 30 minutes. Allow the pressure to release naturally.

VARIATION 2 **Ham Hock Luck & Money:** Add a ham hock and omit the salt.

INGREDIENT TIP *If you eat dairy ingredients, use regular butter.*

PER SERVING Calories: 140; Total fat: 2g; Total carbs: 23g; Sugar: 1g; Protein: 9g; Fiber: 6g; Sodium: 260mg

Prep time: 10 minutes

Cook time: 30 minutes

POT

6 cups peeled, cubed butternut squash

2 Gala apples, unpeeled, cored

2 cups Homemade Vegetable Stock (see substitution tip on page 34)

2 garlic cloves, minced

½ teaspoon onion powder

½ teaspoon salt

¼ teaspoon red pepper flakes

⅛ teaspoon freshly ground black pepper

Unsweetened coconut milk (optional)

Velvety Butternut Squash Soup

Vegan I use fresh butternut squash in season and frozen squash the rest of the year. Because the frozen squash is pre-cubed, it is a great shortcut when you are short on time. Either way, the soup is delicious as a hearty lunch or a light dinner with a side salad and toasted bread.

1. In a large stockpot over medium-high heat, combine the butternut squash, apples, stock, garlic, onion powder, salt, red pepper flakes, and black pepper. Bring to a boil, then reduce the heat to low. Cover and cook for 20 minutes, or until the squash and apples are very tender.

2. Remove the pot from heat. Using an immersion blender, blend the soup until smooth. Alternatively, cool the soup and transfer it in batches to a blender or food processor to blend until smooth.

3. Stir in just enough coconut milk (if using) to achieve your desired consistency.

VARIATION **Sweet Potato Soup:** Use 4 cups peeled, cubed sweet potato in place of the butternut squash. Omit the apples. Add ¼ teaspoon of ground cinnamon.

INGREDIENT TIP *If you eat poultry, use Homemade Chicken Stock (page 34) for a heartier flavor.*

PER SERVING Calories: 82; Total fat: 0g; Total carbs: 21g; Sugar: 9g; Protein: 4g; Fiber: 1g; Sodium: 295mg

CHAPTER 9

Pasta & Grains

Italy may be the first place that comes to mind when someone mentions pasta; nevertheless, pasta is the number one favorite food all over the world. The recipes in this chapter are a great example of why that is true. Pasta is versatile, it pairs with nearly any flavors you can dream up, and it stores well. It's also an affordable option, even when it comes to buying the gluten-free variety.

The Jovial brand is my top pick for gluten-free pasta, and it's what I use in these recipes. I've tried every gluten-free pasta I could find in my local markets and online, and Jovial wins for taste and texture. It works in cold dishes like BLT Bow Tie Pasta Salad (page 114) and holds up equally well in hot, pressure cooked meals such as my Pressure Cooker Vegan Mac 'n Cheese (page 115).

Prep time: 10 minutes

Cook time: 15 minutes

12 ounces sliced uncured bacon (preservative-free)

12 ounces gluten-free bow tie pasta

4 tablespoons Homemade Ranch Seasoning (page 33)

4 tablespoons mayonnaise

4 tablespoons unsweetened coconut milk

1 large tomato

1 romaine heart

BLT Bow Tie Pasta Salad

Dairy-free This simple salad is a crowd-pleaser. It's great as a side dish with grilled chicken or fish, or as a meal on its own. Its leftovers make the best brown-bag lunches. Need a side dish to contribute to a summer barbecue? Look no further.

1. Preheat the oven to 400°F.

2. Place the bacon in a single layer, but not touching, on a large, rimmed baking sheet. Bake for 15 minutes, or until crisp. Transfer to a paper towel–lined plate to drain and cool.

3. While the bacon cooks, prepare the pasta according to the package directions. Drain and rinse under cold water. Transfer to a large serving bowl and refrigerate.

4. In a small bowl, whisk together the ranch seasoning, mayonnaise, and coconut milk.

5. Dice the tomato and chop the romaine into bite-size pieces. Crumble the bacon.

6. Pour the dressing over the chilled pasta and gently stir to coat. Add the tomato, romaine, and bacon crumbles. Stir gently and serve, or chill until ready to serve.

VARIATION **Caribbean Mango Pasta Salad:** Omit the dressing, tomato, bacon, and romaine. Add 1 cup of chopped red bell pepper, 1 cup of diced mango, 2 tablespoons of chopped fresh cilantro, ½ tablespoon of minced jalapeño pepper, and 1 teaspoon of grated lime zest. In a small bowl, whisk together the juice of 1 lime, 1 tablespoon of honey, ½ teaspoon of ground cumin, and ½ teaspoon of grated fresh gingerroot. Toss the dressing with the pasta, then gently toss with the vegetables and mango.

INGREDIENT TIP *Use ¼ to ½ cup of your favorite bottled gluten-free ranch dressing if you don't want to make your own.*

PER SERVING Calories: 331; Total fat: 21g; Total carbs: 25g; Sugar: 2g; Protein: 10g; Fiber: 3g; Sodium: 464mg

Prep time: 5 minutes

Pressure cooking time: 10 minutes

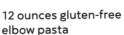
ING MIN POT

12 ounces gluten-free elbow pasta

1 (14-ounce) can full-fat coconut milk

3½ cups water

¼ cup dairy-free butter

6 slices (about 4 ounces) dairy-free Cheddar cheese

1 cup dairy-free mozzarella shreds

1 teaspoon salt

Pressure Cooker Vegan Mac 'n Cheese

Vegan With a serious mac 'n cheese lover in my home, making this classic dish is something I do often. My version streamlines prep and shortens cooking time, which is essential, given how frequently I cook it. This dairy-free version rivals the real deal. It's creamy, comforting, and so easy. Added bonus: It freezes like a dream.

1. Place all the ingredients in the pressure cooker pot in the order listed, then stir.

2. Lock the lid into place. Cook at high pressure for 10 minutes. After cooking, let the pressure release naturally. Unlock and remove the lid.

3. Stir and serve while hot.

VARIATION **Stove-top Mac 'n Cheese:** Prepare 12 ounces of gluten-free elbow pasta according to the package directions; drain and set aside. In a large saucepan over medium heat, combine 1 (14-ounce) can of coconut milk, ¼ cup of dairy-free butter, 6 slices of dairy-free Cheddar cheese, 1 cup of dairy-free mozzarella shreds, and salt. Stir until the sauce is smooth and the cheese is melted. Add the pasta, stir to warm through, and serve.

SUBSTITUTION TIP *If you eat dairy products, replace the coconut milk with heavy (whipping) cream. Replace the vegan cheese with 2½ cups of shredded cheese of your choice. Cheddar is a good option, especially when mixed with an extra-creamy cheese like Fontina.*

PER SERVING Calories: 370; Total fat: 22g; Total carbs: 41g; Sugar: 3g; Protein: 5g; Fiber: 3g; Sodium: 459mg

SERVES 8
Prep time: 10 minutes
Cook time: 45 minutes

¼ teaspoon coconut oil or avocado oil

12 ounces gluten-free penne pasta

1 (25-ounce) jar pasta sauce or 3 cups Five-Minute Pizza/Pasta Sauce (page 31)

25 ounces (about 3 cups) water

2 cups shredded mozzarella cheese, divided

No-Boil Pasta Bake

Vegetarian This recipe turns a weeknight dinner dilemma into a dream. You can have a delicious, no-fuss baked pasta dinner ready in less than an hour, as long as you have the needed pantry ingredients and a casserole dish. It's every busy parent's dinner wish come true.

1. Preheat the oven to 350°F. Lightly grease a 3-quart casserole dish with the oil.

2. Add the pasta, sauce, water, and 1 cup of mozzarella to the prepared dish. Gently stir to mix. Top with the remaining 1 cup of mozzarella. Bake for 45 minutes, or until the pasta is tender.

VARIATION 1 **Beefed-Up Pasta Bake:** Use a 4-quart casserole dish and add ½ pound of cooked ground beef to the pasta. Bake for 45 minutes.

VARIATION 2 **Pasta Bake with Spinach and Parmesan:** Make the recipe as directed, but only use 1 cup of mozzarella. After 35 minutes, remove the casserole dish from the oven and stir in 3 cups of fresh baby spinach leaves (carefully!), then smooth the top of the pasta to an even layer. Top with ¾ cup of grated Parmesan cheese. Bake for 10 minutes more, or until the Parmesan melts and begins to brown.

ALLERGEN TIP *To make this dish vegan, substitute 2 cups of shredded dairy-free cheese for the mozzarella. I like Daiya mozzarella-style shreds. You may also omit the cheese altogether, if you prefer. The baked pasta is delicious without it.*

PER SERVING Calories: 315; Total fat: 9g; Total carbs: 47g; Sugar: 9g; Protein: 11g; Fiber: 3g; Sodium: 560mg

SERVES 8

Prep time: 10 minutes

Cook time: 50 minutes

POT

¼ teaspoon coconut oil or avocado oil

8 ounces gluten-free spaghetti

2½ cups chopped or shredded cooked chicken

1 cup fresh or frozen broccoli florets

2 cups dairy-free Cheddar shreds

1 (14-ounce) can full-fat coconut milk

1 cup Homemade Chicken Stock (page 34)

½ cup water

½ teaspoon salt

½ teaspoon garlic powder

All-in-One Chicken Tetrazzini

Dairy-free · *Egg-free* My family loves tetrazzini, but because I'm not a fan of boiling pasta, I rarely made it until I created this recipe. Now, it's so easy to layer the ingredients in the pan, top with cooking liquid, set the timer for 1 hour, and take care of other tasks around the house while dinner bakes.

1. Preheat the oven to 375°F. Grease a 3-quart, high-sided baking dish with the oil.

2. Break the spaghetti into thirds and place it in the baking dish. Top with the chicken, broccoli, and cheese.

3. In a medium bowl, whisk together the coconut milk, stock, water, salt, and garlic powder. Pour over the ingredients in the baking dish.

4. Bake, uncovered, for 50 minutes. Let rest for 10 minutes before serving.

VARIATION **Tetrazzini with Peas and Gouda:** Omit the broccoli and Cheddar and substitute with frozen green peas and Gouda.

PER SERVING Calories: 405; Total fat: 23g; Total carbs: 26g; Sugar: 3g; Protein: 23g; Fiber: 2g; Sodium: 454mg

Prep time: 15 minutes

Cook time: 30 minutes

¼ teaspoon coconut oil or avocado oil

8 ounces gluten-free spaghetti

1 (28-ounce) jar pasta sauce, divided

8 ounces cream cheese, at room temperature

1 cup part-skim ricotta or cottage cheese

¼ cup sour cream

½ cup grated Parmesan cheese, divided

¼ cup sliced scallions

1 teaspoon Italian seasoning

1 cup shredded mozzarella cheese

Four-Cheese Spaghetti Casserole

Egg-free · *Vegetarian* When my oldest daughter was a toddler, this was her favorite food. We made it every Wednesday for dinner and enjoyed leftovers for the next day's lunch. This recipe relies on dairy ingredients for the best flavor.

1. Preheat the oven to 350°F. Lightly grease a 9-by-13-inch baking dish with the coconut oil.

2. Cook the pasta according to the package directions. Drain the pasta and transfer it to the baking dish.

3. Pour 1 cup of pasta sauce into the baking dish and stir to coat the pasta.

4. In a medium bowl, mix together the cream cheese, ricotta, sour cream, and ¼ cup of Parmesan cheese and stir until smooth. Stir in the scallions and Italian seasoning.

5. Spread the cream cheese mixture carefully over the pasta. Top it with the remaining pasta sauce. Sprinkle the mozzarella and remaining ¼ cup of Parmesan cheese over the top. Bake for 40 minutes.

VARIATION 1 **Spaghetti Casserole with Meat Sauce:** Brown ½ pound of ground grass-fed beef on the stove top and add it to the pasta sauce.

VARIATION 2 **Spaghetti Squash Casserole:** Substitute about 4 cups of cooked spaghetti squash for the pasta for a low-carb dish.

PER SERVING Calories: 292; Total fat: 15g; Total carbs: 29g; Sugar: 4g; Protein: 11g; Fiber: 1g; Sodium: 458mg

Prep time: 10 minutes

Cook time: 15 minutes

MIN

8 ounces gluten-free spaghetti

½ cup extra-virgin olive oil, plus ½ tablespoon

1 cup diced tomato

Juice of 1 lemon

½ cup finely chopped yellow onion

3 tablespoons chopped fresh basil

2 tablespoons capers

½ teaspoon salt

¼ teaspoon freshly ground black pepper

4 (4-ounce) tilapia fillets

Pasta with Tilapia Matecumbe

Dairy-free · *Egg-free* Matecumbe is a place in the Florida Keys, and the name also refers to a particular preparation of fish done in that area. It is my favorite way to enjoy fresh fish, and this recipe is my interpretation of the dish. Mahi-mahi, grouper, snapper, and hogfish are commonly used in the Keys, but the preparation is just as delicious with an easier-to-find, budget-friendly fish like tilapia.

1. Preheat the broiler.

2. Prepare the pasta according to the package directions. Drain and toss with ½ tablespoon of olive oil. Set aside.

3. In a small bowl, stir together the tomato, lemon juice, onion, the remaining oil, basil, capers, salt, and pepper.

4. Place the fish in a broiler-safe baking dish that is at least 2 inches deep and will accommodate the fish fillets in a single layer. Broil for 3 minutes. Carefully turn over each fillet. Pour the tomato mixture over the fillets. Place under the broiler for about 5 minutes, or until the sauce is heated and the fish is cooked through.

5. Divide the pasta between 4 pasta bowls. Top with the fish and sauce. Serve hot.

VARIATION **Vegan Matecumbe:** Substitute thick slices of eggplant for the fish. Brush the eggplant with oil and broil for 3 minutes per side, then top with the sauce and broil until the eggplant is tender.

INGREDIENT TIP *If you can't find capers, substitute ¼ cup of minced green olives.*

PER SERVING Calories: 561; Total fat: 32g; Total carbs: 48g; Sugar: 2g; Protein: 26g; Fiber: 2g; Sodium: 461mg

Prep time: 10 minutes

Cook time: 45 minutes

5
ING

¼ teaspoon coconut oil or avocado oil

15 ounces part-skim ricotta cheese

8 ounces hummus

1 (7-ounce) box gluten-free manicotti shells

1 (26-ounce) jar pasta sauce

12 ounces water

8 ounces provolone cheese, sliced

Cheesy Hummus-Filled Manicotti

Egg-free · Vegetarian Hummus may seem like an odd choice for manicotti filling, but it lends a bright flavor and creamy, ricotta-like texture to pasta dishes. In this recipe, there's no boiling the pasta, so the prep is fast. The manicotti cooks during baking. Once you remove the dish from the oven, allow it to sit for 20 minutes before digging in so the liquid has time to absorb completely.

1. Preheat the oven to 375°F. Grease a 9-by-13-inch glass baking dish with the oil.

2. In a medium bowl, combine the ricotta and hummus until smooth. Place the mixture into a piping bag or a large plastic food storage bag.

3. Snip the corner from the bag and pipe the filling into the uncooked manicotti shells. Place the shells in the baking dish in a single layer.

4. Pour the pasta sauce and water over the filled shells. Top with the provolone slices.

5. Bake for 45 minutes. Let the manicotti sit for 20 minutes before serving.

VARIATION **Dairy-Free Hummus-Filled Manicotti:** Skip the ricotta and use 3 (8-ounce) containers of hummus to fill the manicotti. Top with dairy-free cheese slices before baking.

INGREDIENT TIP *There are usually 16 manicotti shells in a 7-ounce box. I usually have 2 shells left over without filling. I place the empty shells in the baking dish to cook with the others.*

PER SERVING Calories: 464; Total fat: 21g; Total carbs: 43g; Sugar: 8g; Protein: 26g; Fiber: 5g; Sodium: 883mg

Prep time: 10 minutes

Cook time: 40 minutes

1 (26-ounce) jar
pasta sauce

1 large zucchini,
cut into cubes

2 cups peeled and grated
sweet potatoes

1 pound boneless,
skinless chicken
breast strips

8 ounces gluten-free
penne pasta

1 tablespoon
dairy-free butter

Pasta with Chicken in Ratatouille-Style Sauce

Dairy-free • ***Egg-free*** This recipe is a shortcut ratatouille with chicken served over pasta. Just use pasta sauce from a jar (I like Dave's Gourmet brand) and add veggies and boneless, skinless chicken strips. It cooks on the stove top in less than an hour, with no added liquids or seasonings. This dish is all flavor.

1. In a large stockpot over medium-high heat, combine the pasta sauce, zucchini, sweet potatoes, and chicken. Cover and cook until the chicken is tender and cooked through, about 40 minutes.

2. Meanwhile, cook the pasta according to the package directions. Drain and return it to the pot. Add the butter and toss to coat.

3. When the chicken is cooked through, stir the sauce, shredding the chicken slightly with a fork. Divide the pasta between serving bowls and spoon the sauce over it.

VARIATION **Pasta with Chicken, Cauliflower, and Mushrooms:** Substitute chopped onion for the zucchini and riced cauliflower for the sweet potato, and add mushrooms or other veggies of your choice.

INGREDIENT TIP *Some pasta sauces come in a 28-ounce jar, which will work just as well with no need to alter the recipe.*

PER SERVING Calories: 307; Total fat: 4g; Total carbs: 48g; Sugar: 6g; Protein: 22g; Fiber: 5g; Sodium: 491mg

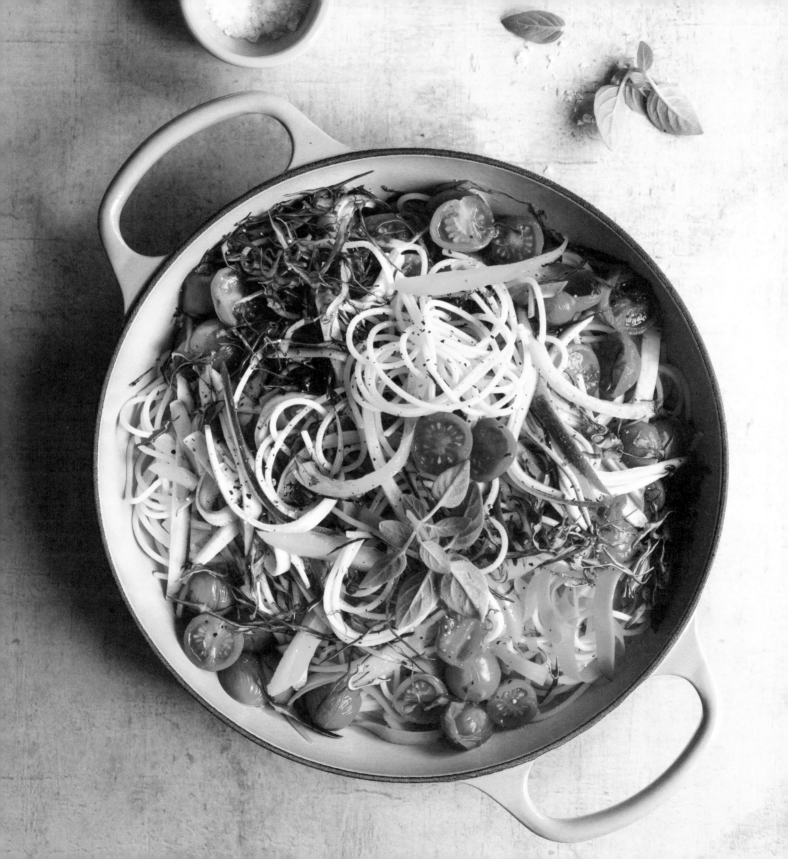

Prep time: 15 minutes

Cook time: 15 minutes

MIN

8 ounces gluten-free spaghetti

2 tablespoons coconut oil or avocado oil

2 cups julienned zucchini

2 cups cherry tomatoes, halved

1 cup carrot ribbons

1 cup yellow bell pepper strips

2 garlic cloves, minced

¼ teaspoon salt

⅛ teaspoon freshly ground black pepper

½ cup white wine

¼ cup finely grated Parmesan cheese

2 tablespoons unsalted butter

½ cup shredded red cabbage

Fresh parsley or basil, for garnish

Farmers' Market Pasta Skillet

Egg-free • *Vegetarian* It doesn't get any easier than this market-fresh feast. You can choose your veggies based on what is fresh and in season. Then you just need to assemble the sauce while the pasta cooks. Add some fresh baked bread (page 191) and dinner is on the table for all to enjoy.

1. Cook the spaghetti according to the package directions; drain and set aside.

2. In a large, deep skillet, heat the oil over medium-high heat. Add the zucchini, tomatoes, carrot, and bell pepper and cook for 5 to 7 minutes, until just becoming tender. Add the garlic, salt, and black pepper and cook for 1 minute.

3. Add the wine, Parmesan, and butter and stir to create the sauce. Add the drained pasta and cabbage and stir to coat.

4. Serve garnished with fresh parsley or basil.

VARIATION **Caponata Pasta:** Substitute cubed eggplant for the zucchini and sliced red onion for the carrot, and omit the bell pepper and cabbage. Add ½ cup of golden raisins and 1 tablespoon of capers. Substitute olive oil for the butter in the sauce. Garnish with ½ cup of sliced black olives and fresh basil leaves.

PER SERVING Calories: 423; Total fat: 15g; Total carbs: 60g; Sugar: 9g; Protein: 10g; Fiber: 6g; Sodium: 328mg

Prep time: 15 minutes

Cook time: 10 minutes

2 ounces gluten-free spaghetti

1 large avocado, chopped

4 tablespoons dairy-free milk, divided

½ cup fresh flat-leaf parsley leaves

¼ cup fresh dill leaves

1 garlic clove

½ teaspoon salt

¼ teaspoon freshly ground black pepper

2 small zucchini, ends trimmed

Zucchini & Pasta with Creamy Herb Sauce

Vegan If you love pasta but want to cut back on carbs, this recipe is a great start. It's also how I encouraged my family to start eating spiral-cut zucchini noodles, or "zoodles." If you don't have a spiral slicer, use your vegetable peeler to cut the zucchini into thin ribbons, or julienne them. Any way you slice it, it's delicious.

1. Cook the pasta according to the package directions. Drain and return to the cooking pot.

2. While the pasta cooks, place the avocado, 2 tablespoons of milk, the parsley, dill, garlic, salt, and pepper in the bowl of your food processor. Process until smooth. If needed, add the remaining milk to thin the sauce.

3. Spiral-slice the zucchini and add it to the pot with the pasta. Add the herb sauce and gently toss to coat the pasta and zucchini. Serve immediately.

VARIATION **Low-Carb Zucchini and Pasta:** Omit the pasta and substitute with 2 additional small zucchini.

INGREDIENT TIP *If you eat dairy products, use regular milk.*

PER SERVING Calories: 364; Total fat: 20g; Total carbs: 44g; Sugar: 3g; Protein: 7g; Fiber: 9g; Sodium: 608mg

SERVES 4

Prep time: 5 minutes

Pressure cooking time: 10 minutes

1 cup Arborio rice

1 small onion, diced

1 tablespoon sunflower oil

2½ cups hot Homemade Vegetable Stock (see substitution tip on page 34) or water

½ teaspoon salt

Almost-Instant Pressure Cooker Risotto

Vegan The pressure cooker makes this beloved, but typically time-consuming, dish cook exceedingly fast when compared with stove top cooking. Consider it a blank slate for your favorite additions, and look forward to a dinner ready in under 30 minutes any night of the week. Adjust the salt in your dish, depending on whether you use low- or no-sodium stock.

1. Place the rice, onion, and oil in the pressure cooker pot. If using a stove-top pressure cooker, sauté the ingredients. If using an electric pressure cooker, press the Sauté/Brown setting and cook the rice and onion for about 5 minutes, stirring occasionally. The rice will become opaque in spots.

2. Add the hot stock and salt. Quickly lock the lid into place. Cook at high pressure for 10 minutes. After cooking, quick release the pressure. Unlock and remove the lid.

3. Stir the rice and serve.

VARIATION 1 **Asparagus Parmesan Risotto:** While the risotto cooks, sauté 1 cup of asparagus tips in ½ tablespoon of butter or oil for 5 minutes. Before serving, stir the asparagus and ½ cup of shaved Parmesan cheese into the risotto. Finish with a few grinds of freshly ground black pepper.

VARIATION 2 **Crispy Risotto Patties:** Form about 3 tablespoons of chilled risotto into a ball and flatten slightly. In a large skillet, fry the risotto patties over medium-high heat for 3 to 4 minutes per side, until crisp and golden. Top with shaved Parmesan cheese and fresh herbs.

PER SERVING Calories: 262; Total fat: 5g; Total carbs: 45g; Sugar: 3g; Protein: 7g; Fiber: 2g; Sodium: 509mg

SERVES 4

Prep time: 10 minutes

Cook time: 25 minutes

POT

1 cup long-grain
white rice

1 tablespoon coconut oil
or avocado oil

2 cups cold water

½ cup diced onion

½ cup drained canned
diced tomatoes

3 tablespoons
tomato sauce

2 garlic cloves, minced

1½ teaspoons minced
jalapeño pepper

1 teaspoon
ground cumin

½ teaspoon salt

Mexican Rice

Vegan Have you ever wondered why the rice at Mexican restaurants is so good? I have the secret! Sauté the rice in oil for a few minutes before you add the water or other cooking liquid. This is called toasting the rice; it lightly splits the grain and leads to lighter, fluffier cooked rice. It also means the grains absorb maximum flavor from the other ingredients.

1. Combine the rice and oil in a large saucepan over medium-high heat. Stir the rice so that every grain is coated with the oil. Stir slowly but consistently, so that it doesn't burn, about 2 minutes. The rice grains will change from translucent to opaque as they heat, and some grains will begin to lightly brown.

2. Once you have lightly browned the rice, quickly add the water, onion, tomatoes, tomato sauce, garlic, jalapeño, and cumin, being careful when you add the liquid to the hot pan, as it will bubble up and steam will rise.

3. Stir quickly to mix, then cover the pan. Reduce the heat to low and cook for 25 minutes. (Note: Stoves vary, so you may need to adjust the cooking time and/or heat level. The first time you make this, check the rice after 20 minutes to make sure it isn't sticking to the bottom of the pan.) The rice is ready when the liquid is absorbed and the rice is tender. It should be on the dry side, not saucy.

VARIATION 1 **Fluffy Plain Rice:** Use the same method of cooking the rice in a small amount of oil, but only add the water or stock and salt. The rice to liquid ratio should be 1:2, so if you have 1 cup of rice, you need 2 cups of liquid.

VARIATION 2 **Coconut Rice:** Replace the water with the liquid portion of canned coconut milk. Add 3 tablespoons of finely grated unsweetened dried coconut, 2 teaspoons of lime zest, and ½ teaspoon of salt. This is an excellent use for leftover coconut water after using the solid portion from a can of coconut milk in another recipe.

MAKE-AHEAD TIP *Mexican Rice or either variation is easy to prepare ahead and freeze. Cool completely and portion the rice into freezer-safe containers. It will last for up to 1 month. Use as needed in soups or stews, or reheat in the microwave for a quick and easy side dish.*

PER SERVING Calories: 144; Total fat: 3g; Total carbs: 27g; Sugar: 1g; Protein: 3g; Fiber: 1g; Sodium: 237mg

SERVES 4

Prep time: 10 minutes

Cook time: 1 hour
15 minutes

POT

¼ teaspoon coconut oil
or avocado oil

1 cup wild rice

1 (14-ounce) can
light coconut milk

½ cup Homemade
Vegetable Stock (see
substitution tip on
page 34)

1½ cups sliced mush-
rooms, such as baby
portobello, cremini, or
oyster, or a mix

1 cup frozen peas

1 tablespoon dairy-free
butter, melted

1 teaspoon salt

½ teaspoon ground sage

½ teaspoon
garlic powder

½ teaspoon
onion powder

⅛ teaspoon freshly
ground black pepper

Wild Rice Casserole

Vegan If "tough" and "chewy" come to mind when you think of wild rice, try this recipe. This dish is creamy and full of flavor, and the rice is tender but not mushy. Sealing the dish with aluminum foil traps the steam inside so the rice cooks perfectly. I like Lundberg Family Farms wild rice because I know it is gluten-free, it's easy to find, and the price is comparable with other brands.

1. Preheat the oven to 375°F. Lightly grease an 8-by-8-inch baking dish with the oil.

2. Combine all the ingredients in the baking dish and stir gently. Cover tightly with aluminum foil.

3. Bake for 1 hour 15 minutes. Remove the foil, stir, and serve while hot or warm.

VARIATION 1 **Apple-Pecan Wild Rice:** Only use ½ cup of mushrooms; omit the peas and garlic powder. Add 1 cup of diced apple and ½ cup of chopped pecans. Bake as directed.

VARIATION 2 **Pub-Style Wild Rice:** Use 1 cup of mushrooms; omit the peas and sage. Add 1 cup of sharp Cheddar cheese cubes and ½ cup of chopped green olives. Bake as directed.

SUBSTITUTION TIP *If you eat dairy, use regular milk and butter in this recipe.*

PER SERVING Calories: 196; Total fat: 8g; Total carbs: 25g; Sugar: 2g; Protein: 6g; Fiber: 3g; Sodium: 479mg

Prep time: 10 minutes

Cook time: 10 minutes

8 ounces rice noodles

¼ cup coconut aminos

1 tablespoon sesame oil

1 teaspoon grated
fresh gingerroot

1 teaspoon rice vinegar

1 teaspoon honey

½ teaspoon
garlic powder

½ teaspoon
onion powder

¼ teaspoon red
pepper flakes

2 teaspoons
sunflower oil

2 cups shredded
vegetables

Chopped fresh cilantro,
for garnish

Sesame seeds,
for garnish

Easy Lo Mein

Dairy-free • *Egg-free* • *Vegetarian* This healthier version of lo mein is a great dish for clearing out the veggie bin. Vegetables like carrots, water chestnuts, scallions, spring peas, chopped broccoli, and shredded cabbage all work well. The sauce is made from coconut aminos, which is lower in sodium than soy sauce and perfect for anyone who loves Asian flavors but cannot eat soy.

1. Place the rice noodles in a large bowl and pour in enough hot water to submerge the noodles. Set aside to soak for 7 to 10 minutes, until tender.

2. In a small bowl, whisk together the aminos, sesame oil, ginger, vinegar, honey, garlic powder, onion powder, and red pepper flakes.

3. Heat the sunflower oil in a wok or large skillet over high heat. Add the vegetables and stir-fry for several minutes, until they are crisp-tender.

4. Drain the noodles and add them to the skillet, along with the sauce. Stir to coat the noodles with the sauce and distribute the vegetables. Serve immediately, garnished with chopped cilantro and sesame seeds.

VARIATION **Chicken Lo Mein:** Add 1 cup of chopped cooked chicken to the pan with the vegetables.

SUBSTITUTION TIP *If you prefer a more traditional lo mein noodle, use gluten-free spaghetti in place of the rice noodles.*

PER SERVING Calories: 419; Total fat: 12g; Total carbs: 70g; Sugar: 6g; Protein: 5g; Fiber: 6g; Sodium: 171mg

Prep time: 10 minutes

Cook time: 10 minutes

8 ounces gluten-free spaghetti

¼ cup tahini

¼ cup coconut aminos or gluten-free soy sauce

1 tablespoon rice vinegar

1 tablespoon honey

1 tablespoon sesame oil

2 teaspoons grated fresh gingerroot

1 garlic clove, minced

¼ teaspoon red pepper flakes

2 cups shredded Napa cabbage

½ cup chopped fresh cilantro

½ cup thinly sliced red onion

Ginger-Tahini Noodles

Dairy-free • ***Egg-free*** • ***Vegan*** Tahini is a paste made from ground sesame seeds. It is easy to find in most grocery stores and is popular in Middle Eastern dishes. Tahini works well with Asian flavors, too, and gives the dressing a perfect consistency to cling to the noodles.

1. Cook the pasta according to the package directions. Drain and return to the cooking pot.

2. In a small bowl, whisk together the tahini, aminos, vinegar, honey, sesame oil, ginger, garlic, and red pepper flakes.

3. Drizzle the dressing over the pasta and add the cabbage, cilantro, and onion. Gently toss to coat, then serve.

VARIATION **Peanut Noodles:** Substitute creamy peanut butter for the tahini. If your peanut butter contains salt and sugar, omit the salt and honey in the dressing.

ALLERGEN TIP *If you cannot eat nut or seed butters, omit the tahini. Whisk together 2 tablespoons of cornstarch and 2 tablespoons of water, then add the other dressing ingredients. Heat in a small saucepan until the mixture bubbles, then remove from heat and add to the pasta.*

PER SERVING Calories: 365; Total fat: 12g; Total carbs: 58g; Sugar: 6g; Protein: 7g; Fiber: 3g; Sodium: 59mg

SERVES 4

Prep time: 10 minutes

Cook time: 15 minutes

1 cup quinoa

½ cup drained and chopped sun-dried tomatoes in oil, plus 2 tablespoons of oil

½ cup cubed fresh mozzarella cheese

¼ cup pitted Kalamata olives, halved

¼ cup chopped fresh basil

½ tablespoon freshly squeezed lemon juice

1 teaspoon dried oregano

½ teaspoon garlic powder

¼ teaspoon salt

¼ cup thinly sliced red onion, for topping

Mediterranean Quinoa

Egg-free • ***Vegetarian*** This is the easiest, most flavor-packed dinner you'll ever make. The salty olives, fresh basil, and tender, fresh mozzarella paired with a tangy, bright dressing transform ho-hum quinoa into something irresistible. If, by chance, you have leftovers, it's the best cold salad, next-day lunch you'll ever pack.

1. Prepare the quinoa according to the package directions.

2. Add the sun-dried tomatoes, mozzarella, olives, basil, sun-dried tomato oil, lemon juice, oregano, garlic powder, and salt to the pot with the quinoa. Stir to combine.

3. Top the quinoa with the red onion and serve.

VARIATION 1 Mediterranean Rice: Substitute rice for the quinoa.

VARIATION 2 Garden-Fresh Mediterranean Quinoa: Omit the sun-dried tomatoes. Add 1 cup of halved cherry tomatoes; 1 cup of peeled, diced cucumber; and ½ cup of chopped green bell pepper.

MAKE-AHEAD TIP *This dish can be made and refrigerated up to 1 day in advance with everything except the mozzarella. Gentle reheating can be done in the microwave. Start with 1 to 2 minutes, stir, and then check the temperature. If it's not warm enough, heat in additional 30-second increments to reach the desired temperature. Add the cheese just before serving and stir.*

PER SERVING Calories: 395; Total fat: 20g; Total carbs: 41g; Sugar: 1g; Protein: 11g; Fiber: 5g; Sodium: 936mg

Prep time: 5 minutes

Cook time: 10 minutes

MIN   POT

2 cups milk

1 garlic clove, minced

2 bay leaves

¼ teaspoon salt

Pinch cayenne pepper (optional)

½ cup gluten-free organic medium-grind cornmeal

½ cup grated Parmesan cheese

Parmesan Polenta

Egg-free • *Vegetarian* Polenta is an Italian dish that is essentially creamy cornmeal porridge. Cornmeal is naturally gluten-free; however, corn is often cross-contaminated with gluten in processing, so be sure to purchase a gluten-free brand. To be sure your corn products are also non-GMO, buy organic.

1. In a 2-quart saucepan over medium-high heat, bring the milk, garlic, bay leaves, salt, and cayenne pepper (if using) to a boil.

2. Slowly add the cornmeal, whisking the entire time to prevent lumps. Cook for 3 to 4 minutes, whisking continuously.

3. Remove from heat and stir in the Parmesan cheese. Serve immediately as is, or top with steamed or roasted vegetables or meat.

VARIATION 1 **Polenta with Mushrooms:** In a large skillet, cook 1 pound of sliced mushrooms with 1 tablespoon of butter and a pinch each of salt and pepper for 4 to 5 minutes, until the mushrooms are tender. Spoon the mushrooms over the polenta to serve.

VARIATION 2 **Garden Polenta Bowl:** Top the polenta with a dollop of hummus, ¼ of a diced avocado, 2 tablespoons of diced tomato, 2 tablespoons of diced cucumber, and a dollop of Greek yogurt or sour cream. Top with a drizzle of extra-virgin olive oil and chopped fresh basil or parsley.

ALLERGEN TIP *To make dairy-free polenta, use unsweetened coconut milk or another dairy-free milk and dairy-free (or no) cheese.*

PER SERVING Calories: 121; Total fat: 6g; Total carbs: 10g; Sugar: 6g; Protein: 9g; Fiber: 1g; Sodium: 336mg

SERVES 4

Prep time: 15 minutes

Cook time: 25 minutes

¼ teaspoon coconut oil or avocado oil

4 medium bell peppers

2 cups cooked quinoa

1 cup diced zucchini

1 cup chopped fresh spinach leaves

1 cup chopped artichoke hearts

1 cup shredded mozzarella cheese

¼ cup mayonnaise

1 teaspoon garlic powder

½ teaspoon onion powder

½ teaspoon salt

¼ teaspoon red pepper flakes

Spinach, Artichoke & Quinoa–Stuffed Peppers

Vegetarian If you love spinach-artichoke dip, you'll love these stuffed peppers. You get a hint of the dip with a healthy dose of protein-packed quinoa. Leftovers are good for the next day's lunch, too.

1. Preheat the oven to 350°F. Lightly grease an 8-by-8-inch baking dish with the oil.

2. Slice off the tops of the peppers and remove and discard the seeds and inner white membranes. Stand the peppers in the baking dish, top-side up.

3. In a large bowl, combine the quinoa, zucchini, spinach, artichokes, mozzarella, mayonnaise, garlic powder, onion powder, salt, and red pepper flakes. Mix well. Spoon the filling into the peppers.

4. Bake for 25 minutes and serve hot.

VARIATION **Mediterranean Quinoa Peppers:** Cook the Mediterranean Quinoa (page 131) and use it to stuff the peppers.

ALLERGEN TIP *Substitute dairy-free cheese for the mozzarella and use vegan mayonnaise in place of the mayo.*

PER SERVING Calories: 247; Total fat: 9g; Total carbs: 36g; Sugar: 8g; Protein: 9g; Fiber: 6g; Sodium: 561mg

Prep time: 20 minutes

Cook time: 30 minutes

¼ teaspoon coconut oil or avocado oil

2 large eggs

½ cup pumpkin purée

2½ cups Homemade Chicken Stock (page 34)

2 cups purity protocol oats

½ cup diced carrot

½ cup diced celery

½ cup diced onion

1 teaspoon baking powder

2 tablespoons sunflower oil

1 teaspoon ground sage

½ teaspoon garlic powder

½ teaspoon salt

Savory Baked Oatmeal

Dairy-free If you think oatmeal is just for breakfast, think again! This savory version reminds me of the pan dressing that we eat at Thanksgiving. Fortunately, this is so easy that you can make it any day of the year. It's delicious on its own or as a side dish with roasted chicken.

1. Preheat the oven to 350°F. Lightly grease an 8-by-8-inch baking dish with the oil.

2. In a large bowl, whisk the eggs. Add the pumpkin purée and stock, and whisk to combine.

3. Add the oats, carrot, celery, onion, baking powder, sunflower oil, sage, garlic powder, and salt. Stir to blend.

4. Pour the mixture into the baking dish. Bake for 30 minutes. Let sit for 10 minutes before serving.

VARIATION **Savory Baked Quinoa:** Substitute quinoa flakes for the oats.

MAKE-AHEAD TIP *This dish can be baked up to 2 days ahead. Cover tightly and refrigerate.*

PER SERVING Calories: 226; Total fat: 12g; Total carbs: 21g; Sugar: 3g; Protein: 10g; Fiber: 4g; Sodium: 827mg

Prep time: 15 minutes

Cook time: 15 minutes

1 tablespoon avocado oil or coconut oil

2 cups cooked rice, of your preference

½ cup finely chopped onion

½ cup julienned carrots

½ cup frozen green peas

3 garlic cloves, minced

1 large egg, beaten (optional)

½ cup bean sprouts

½ cup sliced scallions

3 tablespoons gluten-free soy sauce or coconut aminos

2 tablespoons sesame oil

¼ teaspoon red pepper flakes (optional)

Vegetable Fried Rice

Dairy-free · ***Egg-free*** · ***Vegan*** This is my favorite use for leftover rice. In fact, when I cook rice for another meal, I make extra to ensure there are leftovers to use for this fried rice recipe. It is one of my "clean out the fridge" dishes, because nearly any veggies you have on hand will work. That makes it both delicious and different every time.

1. In a wok or large, deep skillet over high heat, warm the avocado oil. Add the cooked rice, breaking up any clumps by using a fork to flatten and separate them. Stir the rice into the oil until the grains are completely separated.

2. Add the onion, carrots, and peas, stirring them into the rice, and cook for 5 minutes. Add the garlic and cook, stirring, for 1 minute more.

3. Push the rice to one side of the skillet, leaving a small clear area to cook the egg (if using). Pour the egg into the pan and scramble it with a spoon or spatula. Stir the cooked egg into the rice and vegetables.

4. Add the sprouts and scallions, then drizzle the soy sauce and sesame oil over the rice. Stir to coat. Stir in the red pepper flakes (if using). Serve hot.

VARIATION **Pork Fried Rice:** Cook 8 ounces of finely chopped bacon in the skillet before adding the rice. Reduce the avocado oil to ½ tablespoon.

MAKE-AHEAD TIP *Keep 2-cup portions of cooked rice and ½-cup portions of pre-chopped vegetables in the freezer so you can put this meal together in minutes.*

PER SERVING Calories: 249; Total fat: 11g; Total carbs: 33g; Sugar: 3g; Protein: 5g; Fiber: 3g; Sodium: 39mg

CHAPTER 10

Meatless Mains & Seafood

Whether you're reducing your meat intake, upping your fish and shellfish intake for health reasons, or expanding your culinary horizons, this chapter is perfect for you. Recipes like Mock Chicken Salad (page 141) use familiar concepts with plant-based ingredients. In other cases, it's those tried-and-true meals that draw the family to the table. Who can resist a piping hot slice of pizza loaded with veggies and cheese?

Lentils, quinoa, nuts, and seeds are excellent sources of plant-based protein. Seafood is high in protein and contains heart-healthy omega-3 fatty acids, too.

Use cooking techniques like grilling, pan-searing, and broiling to add even more flavor to your meals. Adding herbs and spices to your meat-free dishes keeps them interesting and exciting. The flavors of Indian and Asian cuisines work especially well in meatless dishes.

Prep time: 20 minutes

Cook time: 30 minutes

FOR THE VEGETABLES

¼ teaspoon coconut oil
or avocado oil

½ tablespoon sunflower
oil, divided

3 cups chopped
mushrooms

1 cup fresh or frozen
white or yellow
corn kernels

1 cup fresh or frozen
green peas

1 large onion, diced

2 cups shredded carrots

1 cup diced celery

½ teaspoon salt

⅛ teaspoon freshly
ground black pepper

½ cup unsalted
Homemade Vegetable
Stock (see substitution
tip on page 34)

All-Vegetable Shepherd's Pie

Vegan This recipe uses mushrooms in place of the ground lamb or beef found in traditional shepherd's pie. I like a variety of cremini, portobello, and shiitake for a range of earthy flavors. Feel free to use your favorites, or whatever you have on hand.

1. Preheat the oven to 400°F. Grease a 9-by-13-inch glass baking dish with the coconut or avocado oil.

2. Heat the sunflower oil in a large stockpot over medium-high heat. Add the mushrooms, corn, peas, onion, carrots, celery, salt, and pepper and cook until tender, about 8 minutes.

3. Add the stock a little at a time, enough to create steam but not so much that the vegetables are swimming in liquid. Once the last amount of stock is added, cover the pot to steam the veggies, about 10 minutes. Most of the liquid will cook away. When the vegetables are tender, transfer them to the baking dish.

4. Make the sauce by using the same pot you just cooked the vegetables in. Whisk together the stock, cornstarch, onion powder, and garlic powder until smooth. Cook over medium-high heat until the mixture bubbles and thickens, about 5 minutes. Pour the sauce over the vegetables.

FOR THE SAUCE

2 cups unsalted Homemade Vegetable Stock (page 34)

3 tablespoons cornstarch

½ teaspoon onion powder

½ teaspoon garlic powder

FOR THE MASHED POTATO TOPPING

3 cups plain mashed potatoes

¼ cup nutritional yeast

3 tablespoons dairy-free butter

1 tablespoon snipped dried chives

½ teaspoon salt

⅛ teaspoon freshly ground black pepper

Unsweetened coconut milk, enough to achieve spreading consistency

6 dairy-free Cheddar cheese slices or 1 cup Cheddar shreds (optional)

5. In a large bowl, make the mashed potato topping by combining all the topping ingredients through the coconut milk. Mix well. Spread over the vegetables. Top with the cheese (if using).

6. Bake for 30 minutes, or until bubbly. Let cool for 15 minutes before serving.

VARIATION 1 **Chicken Shepherd's Pie:** Substitute the same quantity of cooked chicken for the mushrooms. Use chicken stock in place of the vegetable stock.

VARIATION 2 **Sweet Potato–Topped Shepherd's Pie:** Use sweet potatoes in place of white potatoes on either the vegetable or chicken version.

SUBSTITUTION TIP *If you eat dairy products, use real butter and cheese.*

PER SERVING Calories: 304; Total fat: 10g; Total carbs: 46g; Sugar: 7g; Protein: 13g; Fiber: 7g; Sodium: 609mg

SERVES 6

Prep time: 20 minutes

Cook time: 20 minutes

POT

1 Pizza Crust
(page 29), unbaked

1 cup Five-Minute Pizza/
Pasta Sauce (page 31)

1 cup shredded
mozzarella cheese

1 cup shredded
Gouda cheese

1 cup grape tomatoes,
halved

½ cup thinly sliced
red onion

¼ cup sliced black olives

½ tablespoon
extra-virgin olive oil

1 teaspoon
Italian seasoning

Veggie Pizza

Egg-free · ***Vegetarian*** I use a 9-by-13-inch baking sheet with a 1-inch rim for this recipe, but you can also use a 12-inch round pizza pan. My family likes a good amount of sauce, so we use 1 full cup, but feel free to reduce the amount, if you prefer. Change the vegetables according to what's on hand and experiment with different cheeses for variety.

1. Preheat the oven to 500°F.

2. Press the dough into a 9-by-13-inch rimmed baking sheet. Bake for 10 minutes.

3. Spread the sauce across the top of the dough. Add the mozzarella and Gouda evenly over the sauce. Top with the tomatoes, onion, and olive slices.

4. Bake for 10 minutes more, or until the cheese is melted and the veggies are tender. Drizzle the olive oil and Italian seasoning over the top, and serve.

VARIATION **Cold Veggie Pizza:** Bake the pizza crust for 12 to 15 minutes, until cooked through. Brush the crust with ½ tablespoon of extra-virgin olive oil and sprinkle with 1 teaspoon of Italian seasoning. In a small bowl, combine 8 ounces of room-temperature cream cheese with 2 tablespoons of mayonnaise or sour cream. Spread across the pizza crust. Top with your choice of raw or cooked vegetables and grated cheese. Press the toppings into the cream cheese mixture, then slice and serve.

ALLERGEN TIP *If you do not eat dairy, substitute dairy-free cheese for the regular cheese. Tossing dairy-free shreds with a little nutritional yeast and oil gives them a more cheese-like taste and consistency.*

PER SERVING Calories: 312; Total fat: 11g; Total carbs: 41g; Sugar: 4g; Protein: 10g; Fiber: 4g; Sodium: 488mg

SERVES 4

Prep time: 10 minutes

COOK   MIN

1 (15-ounce) can chick-peas, drained and rinsed

½ cup finely diced celery

¼ cup finely diced onion

¼ cup chopped sweet or dill pickle

¼ cup shredded apple

2 scallions, thinly sliced

¼ cup vegan mayonnaise

½ tablespoon Dijon mustard

½ teaspoon garlic powder

½ teaspoon dried dill

¼ teaspoon salt

¼ teaspoon freshly ground black pepper

Mock Chicken Salad

Vegan If you love the creamy crunch of chicken salad sandwiches, give this chickpea salad a try. It's terrific as soon as you make it, but when I have the willpower, I mix it and chill it for at least an hour before serving. It gives the flavors time to blend, and it tastes even better cold. Bake a loaf of Top 8–Free Sandwich Bread (page 191) for sandwiches!

1. Place the chickpeas in the bowl of a food processor. Pulse 4 or 5 times to break them down slightly. Do not overprocess.

2. In a large bowl, combine the chickpeas, celery, onion, pickle, apple, scallions, mayonnaise, mustard, garlic powder, dill, salt, and pepper. Stir well. Serve on sandwiches or in lettuce wraps.

VARIATION 1 **Real Chicken Salad:** Substitute 1½ cups chopped cooked chicken for the chickpeas.

VARIATION 2 **Lentil Chickpea Salad:** For added creaminess, substitute ½ cup of cooked red lentils for half the chickpeas.

INGREDIENT TIP *If you are not vegan, use any mayonnaise you prefer.*

PER SERVING Calories: 196; Total fat: 7g; Total carbs: 32g; Sugar: 2g; Protein: 7g; Fiber: 6g; Sodium: 767mg

Prep time: 5 minutes, plus 1 hour to marinate

Cook time: 10 minutes

ING POT

2 portobello mushroom caps

2 tablespoons avocado oil

1 tablespoon coconut aminos or gluten-free soy sauce

½ teaspoon garlic powder

Grilled Portobello Mushroom Burgers

Vegan I make two of these giant mushroom caps when we have them because only two of us love mushrooms. But you can easily double the recipe if needed. Serve the grilled 'shrooms sliced over Almost-Instant Pressure Cooker Risotto (page 125) or on a gluten-free bun piled high with your favorite burger fixings.

1. Using a spoon, scrape the black gills from the underside of the mushroom caps. Rinse under cool water and pat dry.

2. Place the mushrooms in a shallow container or a large zip-top plastic bag. Add the oil, aminos, and garlic powder. Toss to coat the mushrooms. Seal the container and let the mushrooms marinate for at least 1 hour, or refrigerate to marinate overnight.

3. Preheat the grill to high.

4. Shake off any excess marinade and place the mushrooms on the grill. Grill for about 5 minutes per side, until the mushrooms become tender and slightly charred at the edges.

VARIATION 1 **Balsamic Mushrooms:** Substitute balsamic vinegar for the aminos or soy sauce and add ¼ teaspoon of salt.

VARIATION 2 **Oven-Baked Mushrooms:** After marinating, place the drained mushrooms in a baking dish and bake in a preheated 425°F oven for about 20 minutes, or until cooked to your desired tenderness.

PER SERVING Calories: 51; Total fat: 2g; Total carbs: 7g; Sugar: 2g; Protein: 2g; Fiber: 2g; Sodium: 148mg

Prep time: 20 minutes

Cook time: 30 minutes

¼ teaspoon coconut oil or avocado oil

115 grams (about ¾ cup) Quick Baking Mix (page 26)

⅔ cup dairy-free milk

2 large eggs

1 tablespoon sunflower oil

¼ teaspoon freshly ground black pepper

4 cups thinly sliced mixed fresh vegetables

2 tablespoons chopped fresh chives

2 tablespoons chopped fresh flat-leaf parsley

2 garlic cloves, minced

½ cup grated Parmesan cheese (optional)

Garden Vegetable Casserole

Dairy-free · *Vegetarian* I use a mixture of sweet onions, green cabbage, zucchini, carrots, leeks, and green bell peppers when I make this dish. Change the vegetables according to what's in season or what you have in the refrigerator. You can also change the herbs according to what you have on hand to keep the dish fresh and interesting.

1. Preheat the oven to 350°F. Lightly grease an 11-by-7-inch or 9-by-13-inch casserole dish with the coconut oil.

2. In a large bowl, combine the baking mix, milk, eggs, sunflower oil, and pepper. Stir until smooth.

3. Add the vegetables, chives, parsley, and garlic. Stir to coat the vegetables with the batter.

4. Spoon the mixture into the casserole dish and top with the Parmesan cheese (if using).

5. Bake for 35 to 40 minutes, or until set.

INGREDIENT TIPS *I use organic sunflower oil, but any neutral-tasting oil will work. I do not recommend olive oil in this recipe. If you do not have baking mix handy, use 115 grams (about ¾ cup) of Gigi's Everyday Gluten-Free Flour (page 27), plus 1½ teaspoons of baking powder and ½ teaspoon of salt.*

PER SERVING Calories: 135; Total fat: 3g; Total carbs: 23g; Sugar: 4g; Protein: 5g; Fiber: 4g; Sodium: 109mg

2¼ teaspoons avocado oil or coconut oil, divided

8 (6-inch) gluten-free corn tortillas

1 cup sliced mushrooms

1 cup grated potato

1 cup finely diced zucchini

1 garlic clove, minced

½ teaspoon ground cumin

2 ounces cream cheese

1 cup salsa verde, divided

1 cup shredded Monterey Jack cheese

Mushroom, Potato & Zucchini Enchiladas

Egg-free · *Vegetarian* Cream cheese adds a richness to the filling, and green salsa adds a bright alternative to traditional red enchilada sauce. Serve these with a dollop of sour cream, a side of Ultimate Guacamole (page 58), and lime wedges.

1. Preheat the oven to 350°F. Grease an 11-by-7-inch or 9-by-13-inch baking dish with ¼ teaspoon of oil.

2. Place the tortillas on a microwave-safe plate and cover with a damp paper towel. Microwave the tortillas for about 30 seconds. Leave them in the microwave until ready to use to keep warm.

3. Heat the remaining oil in a large skillet over medium-high heat. Add the mushrooms, potato, and zucchini and cook, stirring, for 8 minutes. Add the garlic and cook for 1 minute. Add the cumin, cream cheese, and ¼ cup of salsa and stir to combine. Remove the skillet from heat.

4. Working with 1 warm tortilla at a time, fill it with the veggie mixture. Fold the tortilla over and around the filling and place it in the baking dish seam-side down. Repeat for each remaining tortilla.

5. Pour the remaining salsa over the enchiladas and top with the cheese.

6. Bake for 30 minutes, until heated through and the cheese is melted.

VARIATION **Enchiladas Rojas:** Substitute gluten-free red enchilada sauce for the salsa verde.

ALLERGEN TIP *For a dairy-free dish, use dairy-free cream cheese and shredded cheese.*

PER SERVING Calories: 349; Total fat: 19g; Total carbs: 32g; Sugar: 6g; Protein: 14g; Fiber: 5g; Sodium: 561mg

SERVES 4

Prep time: 10 minutes

Cook time: 45 minutes

POT

1 (28-ounce) can diced tomatoes

1 (15-ounce) can chickpeas, drained and rinsed

1 cup plain dairy-free yogurt

1 cup thinly sliced sweet onion

1 tablespoon dairy-free butter

4 garlic cloves, minced

1 tablespoon curry powder

½ tablespoon minced fresh gingerroot

½ tablespoon ground coriander

½ tablespoon ground turmeric

½ tablespoon ground cumin

½ teaspoon red pepper flakes

½ teaspoon salt

¼ teaspoon ground cardamom

¼ teaspoon ground cinnamon

½ cup chopped fresh cilantro

Vegan Tikka Masala

Vegan True tikka masala is anything but vegan. It is usually made with chicken in a yogurt curry sauce. This version has the same exotic Indian spices and creamy sauce, but without the dairy—or meat. Instead of chicken, I use chickpeas, and I serve this dish over Coconut Rice (see the second variation on page 127) for a complete meal.

1. Place all the ingredients in a large stockpot. Cover and cook on high heat until the mixture comes to a boil. Reduce the heat to low and simmer for 40 minutes.

2. Serve over rice.

VARIATION 1 **Chicken Tikka Masala:** Substitute 2 cups chopped cooked chicken for the chickpeas.

VARIATION 2 **Sweet Potato Masala:** Add 2 cups of cubed cooked sweet potato.

INGREDIENT TIP *If you eat dairy, use regular butter and yogurt.*

PER SERVING Calories: 282; Total fat: 7g; Total carbs: 47g; Sugar: 11g; Protein: 11g; Fiber: 10g; Sodium: 669mg

Prep time: 10 minutes

Cook time: 25 minutes

¼ teaspoon coconut oil or avocado oil

½ tablespoon sunflower oil

1 cup chopped onion

4 garlic cloves, minced

2 teaspoons ground turmeric

2 teaspoons ground cumin

2 teaspoons ground coriander

½ teaspoon ground nutmeg

4 cups cooked spaghetti squash

5 large eggs

2 tablespoons Gigi's Everyday Gluten-Free Flour (page 27)

1 teaspoon salt

Persian-Spiced Spaghetti Squash Bake

Dairy-free · ***Vegetarian*** Persian is one of my favorite cuisines. This dish is my version of *kuku*, which is like a frittata. I love spaghetti squash, but this is the only way the rest of my family will eat it. For the dairy eaters, I serve a dollop of plain Greek yogurt on the side. Leftovers of this dish are delicious reheated or eaten cold.

1. Preheat the oven to 375°F. Grease a 2-quart baking dish with the coconut oil.

2. Warm the sunflower oil in a large skillet over medium-high heat. Add the onion and cook, stirring often, for 5 minutes. Add the garlic and sauté for 1 minute. Add the turmeric, cumin, coriander, and nutmeg to the skillet and stir to coat the onion. Remove from heat.

3. In a large mixing bowl, combine the spaghetti squash, eggs, flour, salt, and onion. Stir the ingredients, then transfer to the baking dish.

4. Bake for 25 minutes. Let cool for 10 minutes before serving.

VARIATION **Persian-Spiced Pasta Bake:** Use 3 cups of cooked gluten-free pasta instead of the spaghetti squash.

INGREDIENT TIP *If you cook with ghee, substitute ghee for the sunflower oil to give the onion more flavor.*

MAKE-AHEAD TIP *To cook spaghetti squash quickly, cut a medium squash in half and wrap each half in plastic wrap or damp paper towels. Microwave for 8 minutes on high. When cool enough to handle, use a fork to scrape out the squash strands.*

PER SERVING Calories: 164; Total fat: 9g; Total carbs: 13g; Sugar: 2g; Protein: 9g; Fiber: 1g; Sodium: 690mg

Prep time: 20 minutes

Cook time: 50 minutes

4 medium sweet potatoes, scrubbed and dried

1 tablespoon sunflower oil

2 tablespoons melted ghee, butter, or dairy-free butter

1 teaspoon chili powder

¼ teaspoon salt

1 cup grated Monterey Jack cheese or dairy-free cheese, divided

1 (15-ounce) can black beans, drained

1 cup whole kernel corn

½ cup diced tomato

¼ cup salsa verde

Tex-Mex Stuffed Sweet Potatoes

Dairy-free · ***Egg-free*** · ***Vegan***   These loaded sweet potatoes are a filling, fiber-full meal that will win over sweet potato skeptics. If you prebake your sweet potatoes on meal prep day, you'll have a fast and easy weeknight meal that's ready in about 20 minutes.

1. Preheat the oven to 400°F. Line a baking sheet with aluminum foil or parchment paper.

2. Place the sweet potatoes on the baking sheet and drizzle them with the oil. Rub the oil over each potato. Bake for about 40 minutes, or until the potatoes are cooked through. Leave the oven on.

3. While the potatoes bake, mix together the ghee, chili powder, and salt in a small bowl.

4. Carefully split each baked sweet potato lengthwise. Use a fork to fluff the potato flesh. Divide the ghee mixture evenly between the 4 potatoes. Divide ½ cup of cheese, the beans, corn, tomato, and salsa between each potato, layering on the ingredients. Top each potato with the remaining cheese.

5. Bake for 5 or 10 minutes to heat through and melt the cheese.

VARIATION **Italian Stuffed Potatoes:** Substitute white baking potatoes for the sweet potatoes. Substitute Italian seasoning for the chili powder. For toppings, use 1 (15-ounce) can of drained cannellini beans; ½ cup of roasted red pepper; ½ cup of diced tomato; and ½ cup of chopped fresh basil. Substitute mozzarella cheese for the Monterey Jack.

PER SERVING Calories: 508; Total fat: 23g; Total carbs: 53g; Sugar: 8g; Protein: 22g; Fiber: 13g; Sodium: 547mg

Prep time: 20 minutes

Cook time: 30 minutes

1 (9-inch) Pie Crust
(page 37), unbaked

3 large eggs

1 (14-ounce) can light
coconut milk

½ teaspoon salt

⅛ teaspoon freshly
ground black pepper

1 tablespoon cold butter

¼ cup crumbled
goat cheese

1 medium tomato,
thinly sliced

1 avocado, halved,
pitted, peeled, and sliced

Tomato Quiche with Goat Cheese & Avocado

Vegetarian Traditional quiche doesn't include cheese, but I use a small amount here. It gives this quiche a lovely flavor, but it is not essential for a delicious result. If you're dairy-free, just omit it. Be sure to use a standard pie plate for this quiche. A deep-dish pie plate will leave too much empty crust at the top.

1. Preheat the oven to 400°F.

2. Bake the pie crust for 10 minutes. Remove the crust from the oven and reduce the oven temperature to 375°F.

3. In a medium bowl, beat the eggs and milk with a hand mixer or immersion blender until light and frothy. Add the salt and pepper and blend. Pour the filling into the crust.

4. Cut the cold butter into pea-size pieces and drop them over the filling. Add the cheese and tomato slices in a single layer on top of the filling.

5. Bake for 30 minutes, until the filling is puffed and golden on top. Let the quiche cool for 20 minutes. Top with the avocado, slice, and serve.

VARIATION 1 **Quiche Lorraine:** Chop 4 slices of bacon and cook it in a skillet until crisp. Drain on a paper towel–lined plate. Add the bacon to the bottom of the crust. Prepare the filling, adding a pinch of ground nutmeg. Pour into the crust. Omit the cheese, tomato, and avocado.

VARIATION 2 **Fancy Brunch Quiche:** Omit the cheese, tomato, and avocado. Add 1 tablespoon of chopped fresh dill to the filling. After baking and cooling the quiche, top with 4 ounces of thinly sliced smoked salmon, dollops of crème fraîche (about ¼ cup total), and 1 teaspoon of minced capers.

ALLERGEN TIP *For a vegan quiche, use dairy-free butter and omit the goat cheese.*

PER SERVING Calories: 457; Total fat: 30g; Total carbs: 40g; Sugar: 3g; Protein: 8g; Fiber: 6g; Sodium: 268mg

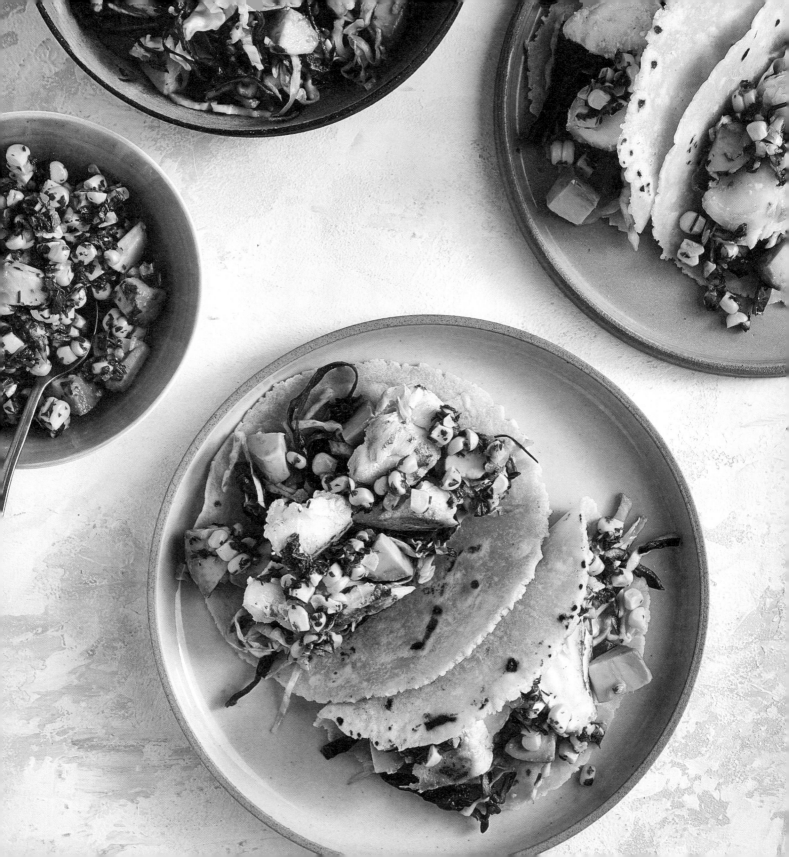

Prep time: 20 minutes

Cook time: 10 minutes

2 tablespoons
sunflower oil

Juice of 1 lemon

½ teaspoon red
pepper flakes

½ teaspoon
ground cumin

¼ teaspoon salt

1½ pounds firm white
fish fillets, like cod

8 Flour Tortillas
(page 36) or gluten-free
corn tortillas

Grilled Fish Tacos

Dairy-free · ***Egg-free*** My favorite way to serve these tacos is with a pile of Cilantro-Lime Slaw (page 73) on top and a side of Corn-Avocado Salsa (page 77). One recipe of my Flour Tortillas (page 36) works perfectly for these tacos, but feel free to use gluten-free corn tortillas if you prefer.

1. In a shallow glass dish, whisk together the oil, lemon juice, red pepper flakes, cumin, and salt. Add the fish and turn once to coat. Set aside to marinate for 15 minutes.

2. While the fish marinates, preheat a grill to medium-high heat.

3. Remove the fish from the marinade, shaking off any excess. Discard the marinade. Grill the fish for about 5 minutes per side, depending on the thickness of the fillets. Grill until the fish flakes when pierced with a fork.

4. Transfer the cooked fish to a clean plate and place a tent of aluminum foil over it. Place the tortillas on the grill for a few seconds on each side to warm.

5. Assemble the tacos by dividing the fish evenly between the tortillas. Serve with the lime wedges and any desired toppings, such as chopped cilantro, diced tomatoes, pico de gallo, shredded cheese, and guacamole.

VARIATION **Shrimp Tacos:** Substitute 1 pound of shrimp for the fish. Thread the shrimp on skewers and grill for 2 to 3 minutes per side.

ALLERGEN TIP *If you do not eat fish or shellfish, substitute an equal amount of chicken breast tenders. Use the same marinade and grill for about 8 minutes per side, or until the chicken is cooked through.*

PER SERVING Calories: 306; Total fat: 10g; Total carbs: 22g; Sugar: 1g; Protein: 33g; Fiber: 3g; Sodium: 277mg

Prep time: 10 minutes

Cook time: 10 minutes

FOR THE SHRIMP

1 pound medium shrimp, peeled and deveined

1 lemon, cut into 4 wedges

¼ cup avocado oil

1 teaspoon dried thyme

¼ teaspoon salt

FOR THE SHORTCUT REMOULADE

½ cup mayonnaise

1 tablespoon Dijon mustard

1 teaspoon hot sauce

1 teaspoon drained capers

½ teaspoon garlic powder

Sheet Pan Shrimp with Shortcut Remoulade

Dairy-free Pair these shrimp with rice or quinoa, or a big salad, and you have dinner in no time. Shrimp prepared this way also work well in shrimp tacos. Just place the shrimp in Flour Tortillas (page 36), load them with Ultimate Guacamole (page 58), and drizzle with the remoulade sauce.

1. Preheat the oven to 400°F. Place a large baking sheet in the oven to preheat it.

2. Place the shrimp in a large bowl and squeeze the lemon wedges over them. Add the lemon wedges to the bowl along with the oil, thyme, and salt. Toss to coat the shrimp.

3. Carefully remove the hot baking sheet from the oven. Place the shrimp and lemon wedges on it in a single layer. Bake the shrimp for 8 to 10 minutes, or until cooked through.

4. While the shrimp bake, make the remoulade in a small bowl by combining all the ingredients. Mix well.

5. When the shrimp are ready, discard the lemon wedges. Serve the shrimp with the sauce on the side.

VARIATION 1 **Red-Hot Apple Shrimp:** Omit the lemon. Add ¼ cup of hot pepper jelly and ¼ cup of apple jelly to the oil, thyme, and salt and stir. Toss with the shrimp before cooking. Omit the remoulade sauce.

VARIATION 2 **Barbecue-Sauced Shrimp:** Reduce the oil to 2 tablespoons and omit the salt. Add ¼ cup of All-American Barbecue Sauce (page 32) and toss with the shrimp before cooking. Serve with the remoulade or additional barbecue sauce.

PER SERVING Calories: 351; Total fat: 25g; Total carbs: 8g; Sugar: 2g; Protein: 25g; Fiber: 0g; Sodium: 710mg

SERVES 4

Prep time: 10 minutes, plus 8 hours to marinate

Cook time: 10 minutes

POT

¼ cup coconut aminos or gluten-free soy sauce

¼ cup melted butter, ghee, or dairy-free butter

¼ cup hot sauce

Chopped rind and juice of 1 lemon

4 garlic cloves, minced

1 teaspoon dried thyme

1 teaspoon dried oregano

1 pound large shrimp, deveined, shells left on

Spicy Southern-Style Shrimp

Dairy-free · *Egg-free* This is a classic Southern dish that is served up family style, accompanied by lemon wedges, additional hot sauce, and lots of toasted (gluten-free) bread. I like to add Cilantro-Lime Slaw (page 73) as a cool, contrasting side dish.

1. In a large zip-top bag or shallow dish with a lid, combine the aminos, butter, hot sauce, lemon rind and juice, garlic, thyme, and oregano.

2. Add the shrimp and toss to coat. Seal or cover and marinate in the refrigerator for 8 to 24 hours.

3. Preheat a grill to high heat.

4. Drain and discard the marinade. Grill the shrimp for 2 to 3 minutes per side, then serve immediately.

VARIATION Spicy Lime-Coconut Shrimp: Omit the hot sauce, thyme, and oregano. Substitute coconut oil for the butter. Add the zest and juice of 1 lime, 1 small seeded and minced jalapeño pepper, and 2 tablespoons of very finely grated dried coconut.

PER SERVING Calories: 255; Total fat: 15g; Total carbs: 5g; Sugar: 0g; Protein: 23g; Fiber: 0g; Sodium: 568mg

Prep time: 20 minutes

Cook time: 20 minutes

4 (6-ounce) salmon fillets

4 teaspoons
sunflower oil

2 teaspoons dried dill

½ teaspoon
garlic powder

¼ teaspoon salt

1 lemon, quartered

4 cherry tomatoes,
halved

4 teaspoons
dairy-free butter

Lemon-Dill Salmon in Parchment

Dairy-free · *Egg-free* I use four parchment bags for this recipe, mainly because it's easier than cutting and folding parchment paper, but you can easily use parchment baking paper to wrap each fillet. Either way, this dish is one of the easiest weeknight meals you'll ever make. It feels fancy, looks beautiful on the plate, and is very healthy.

1. Preheat the oven to 400°F.

2. Rinse the salmon under cold water and pat dry. Rub each salmon fillet with 1 teaspoon of oil. Sprinkle each fillet with dill, garlic powder, and salt. Squeeze a lemon wedge over each fillet and place the lemon on the fish along with 2 cherry tomato halves.

3. Place each fillet in a parchment bag, or in the center of a large piece of parchment paper. Securely wrap the fillets and place the packets in a large baking pan. Bake for about 20 minutes, or until the fish is cooked through.

4. Open the packets and top each fillet with 1 teaspoon of butter. Serve immediately.

VARIATION **Asparagus Butter Salmon:** Omit the oil and dill. Top each piece of salmon with 1 teaspoon of butter before cooking. Add 4 halved asparagus spears to each packet. Top with a few grinds of freshly ground black pepper.

PER SERVING Calories: 330; Total fat: 20g; Total carbs: 4g; Sugar: 2g; Protein: 27g; Fiber: 1g; Sodium: 205mg

SERVES 4

Prep time: 10 minutes

Cook time: 10 minutes

30
MIN

4 (4-ounce) tilapia fillets

2 tablespoons unsalted butter or dairy-free butter, at room temperature

2 teaspoons grated fresh gingerroot

Zest of 1 lime

1 tablespoon freshly squeezed lime juice

½ teaspoon honey

¼ teaspoon salt

⅛ teaspoon freshly ground black pepper

Sheet Pan Tilapia with Ginger-Lime Butter

Dairy-free · *Egg-free* Fish is my go-to weeknight dinner when time is short. It's healthy and cooks in no time. The ginger-lime butter here is perfect for the milder flavor of tilapia. This recipe is also great made with Alaskan cod. I like to serve this over Fluffy Plain Rice (see the first variation on page 127).

1. Preheat the oven to 400°F. Line a baking sheet with parchment paper or aluminum foil.

2. Rinse the fish under cold water and pat it dry. Place it on the prepared baking sheet.

3. In a small bowl, stir together the butter, ginger, lime zest and juice, honey, salt, and pepper. Brush half of the mixture over the fillets. Flip over the fillets and brush the other side with the remaining butter mixture.

4. Bake for about 10 minutes, or until the fish is cooked through and flaky. Serve immediately.

VARIATION **Tilapia with Garlic-Herb Butter:** Omit the ginger, lime, and honey. Prepare the garlic-herb butter first so it has time to chill. Increase the butter to ½ cup and add ½ cup of finely minced fresh herbs (such as parsley, cilantro, tarragon, sage, or basil), 2 minced garlic cloves, ½ teaspoon of salt, and ¼ teaspoon black pepper. Place the butter in the freezer before you place the fish in the oven. Season the fish with salt and pepper and bake as directed. As soon as the fish comes out of the oven, top each fillet with ½ of tablespoon of the cold garlic-herb butter. Serve immediately. Note that this recipe makes more garlic-herb butter than you will need. Refrigerate the leftover butter for up to 1 month or freeze it for up to 6 months.

PER SERVING Calories: 159; Total fat: 7g; Total carbs: 2g; Sugar: 1g; Protein: 22g; Fiber: 1g; Sodium: 259mg

3 (4-ounce) cooked
fish fillets

1 large egg

2 tablespoons
mayonnaise

1 teaspoon capers

½ teaspoon
minced garlic

½ teaspoon
ground cumin

⅛ teaspoon
cayenne pepper

1 tablespoon coconut
oil, divided

Crispy Skillet Fish Cakes

Dairy-free I created this recipe to use leftover fish. If you don't have leftovers, cook the fish according to the cooking method in Sheet Pan Tilapia with Ginger-Lime Butter (page 155), minus the sauce.

1. In a large bowl, shred the cooked fish. Add the egg, mayonnaise, capers, garlic, cumin, and cayenne pepper. Stir well to combine.

2. Place a large skillet over medium-high heat. Add ½ tablespoon of oil.

3. Divide the fish mixture into 4 equal portions. Spoon each one into the hot skillet, patting them down with the back of your spoon and shaping them into patties.

4. Fry for 2 to 3 minutes, then carefully flip each patty with a spatula. Add the remaining oil to the skillet and fry for 2 to 3 minutes more, until crisp.

5. Transfer the fish cakes to a paper towel–lined plate to drain. Serve hot.

VARIATION 1 **Salmon Cakes:** Substitute 12 ounces of canned, drained salmon for the fish.

VARIATION 2 **Vegetarian Patties:** Substitute cooked rice for the fish. Add ¼ cup of grated Parmesan cheese. Omit the capers.

PER SERVING Calories: 173; Total fat: 8g; Total carbs: 2g; Sugar: 1g; Protein: 22g; Fiber: 0g; Sodium: 166mg

Prep time: 15 minutes

Cook time: 10 minutes

1½ tablespoons avocado oil, divided

3 tablespoons drained capers

3 tablespoons cornstarch

½ teaspoon salt

½ teaspoon garlic powder

Zest and juice of 1 lemon

1 pound cod fillets, rinsed and patted dry

2 tablespoons dairy-free butter

Cod with Lemon-Caper Sauce

Dairy-free · Egg-free Cooking capers in oil really brings out their flavor. But be careful not to cook them for too long, as they burn easily. If you're not a fan of their briny flavor, simply omit them from the recipe. Add some chopped fresh dill or parsley over the fish when you serve it instead.

1. Heat ½ tablespoon of oil in a large skillet over medium-high heat. Add the capers and cook for 2 minutes. Transfer the capers to a small bowl.

2. Place the cornstarch, salt, garlic powder, and lemon zest in a large zip-top bag. Toss to combine. Add the fillets, seal the bag, and toss to coat the fish.

3. Place the skillet used to cook the capers back over medium-high heat, and add the remaining 1 tablespoon of oil. When the pan is hot, add the fish, discarding any excess coating. Cook the fillets for 3 to 4 minutes per side, depending on the thickness of the fillets.

4. When the fish is cooked through, add the capers, lemon juice, and butter to the skillet. Swirl the pan to blend the flavors. Turn the fish once. Serve immediately.

VARIATION **Baked Salmon with Lemon-Caper Sauce:** Preheat the oven to 375°F. Place 4 salmon fillets in a baking pan. Season with salt and pepper, and drizzle each fillet with 1 teaspoon of sunflower oil. Bake for 15 to 20 minutes. While the salmon bakes, cook the capers in a skillet as directed. Omit the remaining tablespoon of oil, cornstarch, salt, and garlic powder. Turn off the heat after cooking the capers and add the lemon juice and zest, butter, and 1 minced garlic clove. Spoon the sauce over the cooked fillets.

INGREDIENT TIP *Use real butter if you eat dairy products.*

PER SERVING Calories: 241; Total fat: 12g; Total carbs: 6g; Sugar: 0g; Protein: 27g; Fiber: 0g; Sodium: 604mg

CHAPTER 11

Poultry, Beef & Pork

It's no surprise that chicken is America's favorite protein. It is affordable and adaptable. White or dark meat? Skin on or off? Bone in or boneless? Those are the questions that first come to mind when we consider how we like our bird. I specify what works best on each count.

When it comes to beef, I prefer grass-fed, both for flavor and for its nutritional profile. Serving quality cuts less often and making pricier cuts of meat a side item instead of the main course are effective ways to save money. Make the most of your meat purchases by following the cooking directions so you end up with tender, juicy results every time.

When it comes to pork, look for sales. Summer brings lower prices on shoulder roasts, perfect for making melt-in-your-mouth Slow Cooker Barbecue Pork (page 178), and holidays like Easter and Thanksgiving bring great deals on hams for making Apricot & Mustard–Glazed Ham (page 177).

Prep time: 10 minutes

Cook time: 1 hour
30 minutes

1 tablespoon dried
harissa seasoning

3 tablespoons
extra-virgin olive oil

½ teaspoon salt

1 (4-pound)
whole chicken

1 cup Homemade
Chicken Stock (page 34),
wine, or water

Roasted Harissa Chicken

Dairy-free · Egg-free This recipe calls for dry, ground harissa seasoning, which is a Tunisian spice. You can find it in the ethnic foods section in most grocery stores. Adjust your cooking time according to the size of the chicken you have. Be sure its internal temperature reaches between 165°F and 170°F before removing it from the oven.

1. Preheat the oven to 425°F and have ready a roasting pan with a rack inside.

2. In a small bowl, combine the harissa, oil, and salt into a smooth paste.

3. Rinse the chicken under cold water and pat it dry with paper towels. Place it on the rack in the roasting pan.

4. Gently run your fingers under the skin near the neck area and lift, but do not tear or remove the skin. Distribute half of the harissa mixture under the skin and the other half on top of the skin.

5. Pour the liquid into the pan beneath the chicken. Roast for about 1 hour. During this hour, baste the chicken with the pan juices occasionally, adding more liquid if the pan becomes too dry. For the remainder of the roasting time, about 30 minutes more, do not baste the chicken.

6. Let the chicken rest for 15 minutes. Then transfer it to a platter and carve.

VARIATION 1 **Lemon-Herb–Roasted Chicken:** Omit the harissa and oil. Cut 1 lemon in half and squeeze the juice over the chicken. Place the lemon halves in the cavity along with 6 whole peeled garlic cloves and several rosemary and thyme sprigs. Brush the top of the skin with softened butter and liberally season with salt and pepper.

VARIATION 2 **Barbecue-Roasted Chicken:** Omit the harissa, oil, and salt. Combine ½ cup of All-American Barbecue Sauce (page 32) and 2 tablespoons of melted butter or oil. Brush some under the skin of the breast and the rest over the top of the whole chicken. Baste the chicken several times with more sauce during roasting.

PER SERVING Calories: 495; Total fat: 36g; Total carbs: 1g; Sugar: 1g; Protein: 43g; Fiber: 0g; Sodium: 511mg

Sweet-and-Spicy Ruby-Glazed Drumsticks

Dairy-free · *Egg-free* Dark meat and bone-in chicken are the most flavorful. Add this quick-fix sweet-and-spicy glaze and you're in for a treat. Pepper jelly is usually near the cheese section of most grocery stores. If you've never bought it, trust the recipe and give it a try. Combined with the other ingredients, it creates an irresistible glaze you'll want to use on chicken, pork, and shrimp.

1. Preheat the oven to 400°F. Line a baking sheet with aluminum foil or lightly grease with the oil.

2. Place the drumsticks on the baking sheet.

3. In a small bowl, stir together the tomatoes, pepper jelly, garlic powder, and salt. Spoon 1 tablespoon of glaze over each drumstick.

4. Bake for 30 minutes. Baste the drumsticks generously with more glaze and return to the oven for 10 to 15 minutes more, or until cooked through.

5. If you have leftover glaze, heat it in a small saucepan over medium-high heat just until it boils. Cool slightly and serve on the side with the drumsticks, if desired.

VARIATION **Sweet Glazed Drumsticks:** For something less spicy, substitute an equal amount of apple jelly for the red pepper jelly.

PER SERVING Calories: 536; Total fat: 28g; Total carbs: 31g; Sugar: 30g; Protein: 42g; Fiber: 1g; Sodium: 427mg

Prep time: 20 minutes

Cook time: 45 minutes

1¼ teaspoons coconut oil or avocado oil, divided

2 cups cubed sweet potatoes

½ recipe Pie Crust (page 37), unbaked

2 cups chopped cooked chicken

1 cup frozen green peas

1 cup cooked rice

½ cup minced onion

1 (14-ounce) can light coconut milk

1 cup Homemade Chicken Stock (page 34)

3 tablespoons cornstarch

1 teaspoon dried cilantro

½ teaspoon garlic powder

½ teaspoon salt

⅛ teaspoon freshly ground black pepper

½ tablespoon melted dairy-free butter

Chicken Pot Pie

Dairy-free • *Egg-free* This is traditional chicken pot pie with a tender, flaky, rolled crust top. You will use half of the dough prepared in the recipe for Pie Crust on page 37. Make the full dough amount, use half for this recipe, and freeze the other half for another use or make two pot pies and freeze one.

1. Preheat the oven to 425°F. Grease a 3-quart baking dish with ¼ teaspoon of oil.

2. Place the sweet potatoes in a large roasting pan and drizzle with the remaining oil. Toss to coat. Roast for 20 minutes.

3. While the potatoes roast, roll the pie crust dough into a shape that will fit the prepared baking dish. Set aside.

4. Once the potatoes are done, remove them from the oven and reduce the oven temperature to 375°F. Place the potatoes in the baking dish. Add the chicken, peas, rice, and onion.

5. In a medium bowl, whisk together the milk, stock, cornstarch, cilantro, garlic powder, salt, and pepper. Pour over the chicken and vegetables and stir to combine.

6. Place the pie crust dough over the chicken-vegetable mixture in the baking dish. Use a sharp knife to cut several slits in it. Brush the top of the dough with the butter.

7. Bake for 45 minutes.

VARIATION **Vegetarian Pot Pie:** Replace the chicken with an equal amount of chopped mushrooms and/or additional vegetables. Use vegetable stock in place of the chicken stock.

SUBSTITUTION TIP *If you eat dairy, use dairy milk instead of coconut milk and dairy butter for brushing the crust.*

PER SERVING Calories: 330; Total fat: 5g; Total carbs: 54g; Sugar: 3g; Protein: 14g; Fiber: 3g; Sodium: 298mg

Roasted Lemon Chicken with Potatoes

SERVES 4

Prep time: 15 minutes

Cook time: 40 minutes

POT

4 chicken leg quarters

1 pound petite potatoes

¼ cup avocado oil or coconut oil

Juice and zest of 1 lemon

1 tablespoon dried rosemary

4 garlic cloves, halved

½ teaspoon salt

⅛ teaspoon freshly ground black pepper

Dairy-free · Egg-free An entire meal in one dish is perfect for a Sunday supper or a weeknight meal. The leftovers, if you have any, can be transformed into chicken salad, wraps, or sandwiches, or eaten as is. If you can't find petite potatoes, use small red potatoes and cut them into 1-inch cubes.

1. Preheat the oven to 400°F.

2. Rinse the chicken under cold water and pat dry with paper towels. Place the chicken in a large nonmetal baking dish.

3. Place the potatoes around the chicken pieces.

4. Drizzle the oil and lemon juice over the chicken and potatoes, stirring the potatoes to coat. Top with the lemon zest, rosemary, garlic, salt, and pepper.

5. Roast for 40 to 50 minutes, stirring the potatoes halfway through and spooning some cooking liquid over the chicken. The chicken is done when it reaches an internal temperature of 165°F.

VARIATION 1 **Fajita-Inspired Roast Chicken:** Substitute a lime for the lemon. Omit the rosemary and add 2 teaspoons of ground cumin.

VARIATION 2 **Autumn Chicken Bake:** Use 1 pound of peeled and cubed sweet potatoes in place of the petite potatoes. Add 1 peeled and quartered red onion and 1 medium scrubbed and cubed turnip.

PER SERVING Calories: 396; Total fat: 27g; Total carbs: 20g; Sugar: 2g; Protein: 21g; Fiber: 3g; Sodium: 481mg

¼ teaspoon coconut oil or avocado oil (optional, for greasing)

1 cup gluten-free rice cereal

⅓ cup Homemade Ranch Seasoning (page 33)

¼ cup Quick Baking Mix (page 26)

1 large egg

1 tablespoon sunflower oil

1 pound boneless, skinless chicken breast tenders

Crispy Chicken Strips

Dairy-free While the chicken bakes, I prepare a dipping sauce for these crispy tenders. Simply stir together 2 tablespoons of peach preserves, 1 tablespoon of Dijon mustard, and ¼ teaspoon of garlic powder.

1. Preheat the oven to 425°F. Line a baking pan with aluminum foil or parchment paper. If you use foil, grease it with the coconut or avocado oil.

2. In the bowl of a food processor, combine the cereal, ranch seasoning, and baking mix. Blend until it looks like fine crumbs. Transfer the mixture to a shallow bowl or large plate.

3. In a separate shallow bowl, whisk together the egg and sunflower oil.

4. Dip each chicken tender in the egg mixture, then press all sides into the crumb coating. Place in the baking pan. Repeat with all the chicken tenders.

5. Bake for 25 to 30 minutes, until the chicken is cooked through and the breading is crisp and golden. Serve immediately.

VARIATION **Crispy Oven Fish:** Use the same seasoning and technique with almost any white fish fillets. Reduce the baking time to 10 to 15 minutes, depending on the size and thickness of the fish. Fish should flake with a fork when done.

ALLERGEN TIP *If you cannot eat rice, substitute an equal amount of another crunchy gluten-free food, like potato chips, tortilla chips, or crackers, for the rice cereal.*

PER SERVING Calories: 214; Total fat: 5g; Total carbs: 9g; Sugar: 0g; Protein: 25g; Fiber: 1g; Sodium: 771mg

Prep time: 10 minutes,
plus 8 hours to marinate

Cook time: 15 minutes

1 pound chicken breast,
cut into thin strips

Juice of 1 lime

2 tablespoons
sunflower oil

2 teaspoons
ground cumin

1 teaspoon garlic powder

½ teaspoon salt

Chicken Fajitas

Dairy-free · ***Egg-free*** In the morning, I put the chicken in a bag to marinate so by dinner time it's ready to cook. Make a batch of Flour Tortillas (page 36) and Ultimate Guacamole (page 58) to pair with these flavorful fajitas.

1. Place all the ingredients in a large zip-top bag. Seal and massage the chicken to coat it in the marinade. Marinate in the refrigerator for 8 to 12 hours.

2. Remove the chicken from the marinade, shaking off any excess. Discard the marinade.

3. Place a large skillet over high heat. Lay the chicken strips in the skillet, making sure the pieces are in a single layer. Cook the chicken for about 7 minutes per side, or until cooked through.

VARIATION 1 **All-Veg Fajitas:** Use 1 thinly sliced onion, 2 bell peppers cut into strips, and 8 ounces of sliced mushrooms instead of the chicken. Cook the vegetables in the skillet until tender. Serve with tortillas, guacamole, and hummus.

VARIATION 2 **Steak Fajitas:** Substitute very thinly sliced skirt steak for the chicken. Add 2 tablespoons of gluten-free soy sauce or coconut aminos to the marinade. Cook the steak strips for 3 to 5 minutes, or until cooked through.

PER SERVING Calories: 200; Total fat: 10g; Total carbs: 2g; Sugar: 0g; Protein: 24g; Fiber: 0g; Sodium: 351mg

SERVES 4

Prep time: 15 minutes, plus 4 hours to marinate

Cook time: 22 minutes

POT

4 boneless, skinless chicken breasts

½ cup coconut aminos or gluten-free soy sauce

2 tablespoons honey

1 tablespoon ground turmeric

1 tablespoon sunflower oil

1 teaspoon garlic powder

1 teaspoon ground cardamom

Turmeric-Honey Baked Chicken Breasts

Dairy-free · Egg-free This is a great recipe to double when meal prepping. The chicken is flavorful, tender, and versatile enough to use in a variety of meals. If you aren't a fan of the earthy flavor of turmeric, reduce the amount by half. If you're short on time, use the pressure cooker variation.

1. Place all the ingredients in a large zip-top bag. Seal and turn the bag to coat the chicken. Place the bag on a baking sheet or in a baking dish (in case of leaks) and refrigerate for at least 4 hours or overnight. Alternatively, whisk together the marinade ingredients in a shallow glass dish, then add the chicken, turning to coat. Cover the dish with a tight-fitting lid and refrigerate to marinate.

2. Preheat the oven to 400°F.

3. Place the chicken breasts in a baking dish. Discard the marinade.

4. Bake for 20 to 22 minutes, until the chicken is cooked through and reaches an internal temperature of at least 165°F. Serve immediately.

VARIATION **Pressure Cooker Turmeric and Honey Chicken:** After the chicken marinates, place all the ingredients in the pressure cooker pot. Use the Poultry setting to cook at high pressure for 10 minutes, or manually input or monitor the time yourself. After cooking, let the pressure release naturally before unlocking the lid and serving.

INGREDIENT TIP *You may use an equal amount of pure maple syrup, agave nectar, or granulated sugar for the honey if you prefer.*

PER SERVING Calories: 223; Total fat: 5g; Total carbs: 17g; Sugar: 9g; Protein: 26g; Fiber: 0g; Sodium: 110mg

Prep time: 15 minutes,
plus 8 hours to marinate

Cook time: 10 minutes

1 medium onion, diced

Zest and juice of 1 lime

6 garlic cloves, halved

½ cup apple
cider vinegar

½ cup pineapple juice

¼ cup freshly squeezed
orange juice

¼ cup coconut aminos

¼ cup sunflower oil

1 tablespoon
granulated sugar

1 tablespoon
ground allspice

1 tablespoon
dried thyme

1½ teaspoons
ground sage

1 teaspoon
cayenne pepper

½ teaspoon
ground nutmeg

½ teaspoon
ground cinnamon

½ teaspoon freshly
ground black pepper

2 pounds chicken
breast tenders

Grilled Jerk Chicken Tenders

Dairy-free · Egg-free This is without a doubt my family's favorite chicken recipe. It's on repeat all summer long at our house, and I also use the marinade for vegetables like yellow squash, eggplant, zucchini, and mushrooms. The ingredient list is a bit long, but everything together creates an irresistible flavor.

1. In a shallow glass dish that has a lid, whisk together all of the ingredients except for the chicken breast tenders.

2. Add the chicken and turn to coat. Cover and refrigerate for at least 8 hours or overnight.

3. Preheat the grill to high.

4. Remove the chicken from the marinade, shaking off any excess. Discard the marinade.

5. Grill the chicken for 5 to 7 minutes per side, or until cooked through. The chicken will be very tender, so be careful when turning it. The granulated sugar and the sugars in the fruit juice may cause the chicken to stick to the grill. Serve immediately.

INGREDIENT TIP *If you eat soy, substitute gluten-free soy sauce for the coconut aminos. The chicken will be saltier with the soy sauce.*

PER SERVING Calories: 239; Total fat: 10g; Total carbs: 13g; Sugar: 6g; Protein: 23g; Fiber: 1g; Sodium: 238mg

Prep time: 15 minutes

Cook time: 30 minutes

FOR THE FILLING

¼ teaspoon coconut oil
or avocado oil

2 cups cooked,
shredded chicken

½ cup salsa verde

1 cup black beans

1 cup shredded Cheddar
cheese or dairy-free
cheese shreds

¼ cup chopped
black olives

¼ cup chopped
green olives

¼ cup sliced scallions

4 garlic cloves, minced

FOR THE CRUST

1 cup cornmeal

2 large eggs

½ cup milk or
unsweetened
coconut milk

2 tablespoons
sunflower oil

2 teaspoons
baking powder

½ teaspoon salt

Chicken Tamale Pie

Dairy-free This dish is easy and flavorful. Even if you aren't a fan of olives, give it a try. They cook into the filling and provide a tangy-salty flavor that works well with the cornbread topping. Serve with Ultimate Guacamole (page 58), sour cream (regular or dairy-free), and diced fresh tomato.

1. Preheat the oven to 375°F. Grease an 8-by-8-inch baking dish with the oil.

2. Assemble the filling by stirring together the chicken and salsa in the baking dish. Add the beans, cheese, black and green olives, scallions, and garlic. Stir to combine.

3. Make the crust by whisking together all the ingredients in a medium bowl. Whisk until smooth. Pour the batter evenly over the filling.

4. Put the baking dish in the oven and bake for 30 minutes, until the crust is cooked through in the center.

VARIATION 1 **Bean-Free Tamale Pie:** Substitute the black beans with corn, chopped cauliflower or broccoli, or cubed sweet potatoes.

VARIATION 2 **Southwestern Breakfast Bake:** Replace the chicken with 1 cup browned bulk breakfast sausage. Use ½ cup of corn in place of half the beans. Just before the casserole is done, prepare 4 eggs over easy (or poached) and place one on top of each serving.

PER SERVING Calories: 528; Total fat: 24g; Total carbs: 40g; Sugar: 3g; Protein: 39g; Fiber: 7g; Sodium: 820mg

MAKES 1 (12-INCH) PIZZA

Prep time: 35 minutes

Cook time: 12 minutes

1 Pizza Crust
(page 29), unbaked

5 tablespoons
All-American Barbecue
Sauce (page 32), divided

1 cup diced
cooked chicken

1 cup shredded
Gouda cheese

1 cup shredded
mozzarella cheese

¼ cup thinly sliced
red onion

3 tablespoons chopped
fresh cilantro, for
garnish (optional)

Barbecue Chicken Pizza

Egg-free If you're a fan of the West Coast pizza chain that made this pizza popular, you'll love how easy it is to make. The key to replicating the flavor is the Gouda cheese, so don't skip it. Slice the onions paper thin and add an extra drizzle of barbecue sauce before serving for an extra kick of flavor.

1. Preheat the oven to 500°F. Line a 12-inch round pizza pan with parchment paper.

2. Roll out the pizza dough and place it on the pan. Spread 3 tablespoons of barbecue sauce across the dough. (The dough does not need to be prebaked.)

3. In a small bowl, toss the chicken with the remaining 2 tablespoons of sauce. Place the chicken evenly over the dough.

4. Top the pizza with the Gouda, mozzarella, and onion. Bake for 10 to 12 minutes, until the cheese is melted and the crust is golden. Garnish with fresh cilantro (if using) and serve.

VARIATION 1 **Pesto Chicken Pizza:** Replace the barbecue sauce with pesto, use mozzarella cheese only, and add thinly sliced tomato. Omit the cilantro, and garnish with fresh basil leaves.

VARIATION 2 **Mexican Chicken Pizza:** Replace the barbecue sauce with enchilada sauce; use Monterey Jack and Cheddar cheeses. Add thinly sliced bell pepper and jalapeños to taste.

MAKE-AHEAD TIP *Keep a pizza crust or two in the freezer for when the mood strikes. Thaw the crust at room temperature before using.*

PER SERVING (⅛ pizza): Calories: 278; Total fat: 8g; Total carbs: 36g; Sugar: 3g; Protein: 13g; Fiber: 2g; Sodium: 306mg

Prep time: 5 minutes

Cook time: 15 minutes

¼ teaspoon coconut oil
or avocado oil (optional,
for greasing)

1 pound grass-fed
ground beef

2 tablespoons
minced onion

1 tablespoon
coconut aminos

1 garlic clove, minced

½ teaspoon dried thyme

¼ teaspoon salt

⅛ teaspoon freshly
ground black pepper

Traditional Meatballs

Dairy-free · ***Egg-free*** Make an extra batch of meatballs to freeze so you can always have some handy. There's no real need to add bread crumbs, egg, or other fillers to your meatballs. Use the best-quality beef you can buy, with about 8 percent fat for the best flavor. And don't overcook the meatballs. These are great on their own, in Speedy Beef Stroganoff (page 172), and, of course, in gluten-free spaghetti and meatballs.

1. Preheat the oven to 375°F. Line a baking sheet with aluminum foil or lightly grease it with the oil.

2. In a large bowl, combine the beef, onion, aminos, garlic, thyme, salt, and pepper. Stir well until the mixture is uniform.

3. Shape the meat mixture into 24 meatballs, placing them on the prepared baking sheet.

4. Bake for 15 minutes, or until cooked through.

VARIATION 1 Meatballs in Sauce with Fresh Parsley: Form the meatballs and place them in a large saucepan with a full recipe of Five-Minute Pizza/Pasta Sauce (page 31). Simmer for 25 minutes, or until the meatballs are cooked through. Spoon the meatballs and sauce into a serving bowl and top with ¼ cup of chopped fresh parsley.

VARIATION 2 Sliders: Before cooking, flatten the meatballs into patties on the baking sheet. Bake for 10 to 12 minutes, until cooked through. Use Yeast-Free Muffin Pan Dinner Rolls (page 186) as buns.

MAKE-AHEAD TIP *Prepare the meatballs though step 3. Place them on a baking sheet and freeze solid, about 2 hours. Transfer the frozen uncooked meatballs to freezer bags or airtight containers and freeze for up to 1 month. Take out as many as needed when you're ready to use them. Thaw and cook as desired.*

PER SERVING Calories: 337; Total fat: 28g; Total carbs: 2g; Sugar: 0g; Protein: 18g; Fiber: 0g; Sodium: 227mg

SERVES 4

Prep time: 10 minutes

Cook time: 20 minutes

FOR THE MEATLOAF

¼ teaspoon coconut or avocado oil (optional, for greasing)

1 pound lean grass-fed ground beef

1 large egg

1 tablespoon dried cilantro

1 tablespoon Dijon mustard

½ cup minced onion

½ teaspoon garlic powder

½ teaspoon salt

½ teaspoon smoked paprika

⅛ teaspoon freshly ground black pepper

FOR THE TOPPING (OPTIONAL)

4 tablespoons ketchup

1 teaspoon sugar or honey

¼ teaspoon garlic powder

Mini Meatloaves

Dairy-free When my daughters were younger, they loved meatloaf. The only problem was that it took a long time to bake, so it wasn't an easy weeknight meal. I decided to take my favorite recipe and divide it into mini loaves to slash the baking time. Now it's an anytime meal! These are also great to make ahead and freeze—before or after baking—for quick meals in the future.

1. Preheat the oven to 400°F. Line a baking pan with aluminum foil or lightly grease it with the oil.

2. In a large bowl, combine the beef, egg, cilantro, mustard, onion, garlic powder, salt, paprika, and pepper, and stir until the mixture is uniform.

3. Divide the mixture into 4 equal portions. Shape each into an oval mini loaf and place in the baking pan a few inches apart. Gently press the center area of each oval so it's slightly lower than the outermost edges to ensure even cooking.

4. If making the topping, whisk together all the ingredients in a small bowl. Spread 1 tablespoon of sauce over each mini meatloaf before baking, if desired.

5. Bake for 20 to 22 minutes, until cooked through. Serve hot.

VARIATION 1 **Barbecue-Cheddar Mini Meatloaves:** Add 1 cup of grated Cheddar cheese to the meat mixture before dividing into individual loaves. Use 1 tablespoon of your favorite barbecue sauce as the topping.

VARIATION 2 **Lamb Loaves with Feta and Mint:** Replace half or all of the beef with ground lamb. Add ½ cup of crumbled feta cheese and 1 tablespoon of minced fresh mint leaves to the meatloaf mixture. Skip the topping and sprinkle the loaves with sliced olives (optional).

MAKE-AHEAD TIP *Prepare the meatloaves as directed through step 3 and place them in an airtight freezer-safe container; freeze for up to 1 month. Thaw, make the topping if desired, then bake as directed.*

PER SERVING Calories: 278; Total fat: 14g; Total carbs: 2g; Sugar: 1g; Protein: 32g; Fiber: 1g; Sodium: 428mg

Prep time: 30 minutes

Cook time: 40 minutes

8 ounces gluten-free
egg noodles

1 recipe Traditional
Meatballs (page 170)

1 recipe Creamy
Dairy-Free Mushroom
Soup (page 104)

4 tablespoons sour
cream (omit if dairy-free)

2 tablespoons chopped
fresh flat-leaf parsley

Speedy Beef Stroganoff

Dairy-free This recipe includes two other recipes from this book.
If you prep ahead and have meatballs in the freezer, it makes a fast
weeknight dinner. If not, the meatballs only take about 15 minutes
to make, and they can cook while you prepare the pasta and
mushroom soup.

1. Cook the noodles according to the package directions. Drain and return
them to the cooking pot. Cover to keep warm.

2. Prepare the meatballs and mushroom soup while the noodles cook.
You will need ½ cup of soup per person for this recipe, so you will have
some left over for another use.

3. To serve, divide the noodles between 4 shallow bowls and top with
the meatballs.

4. In a small bowl, stir the sour cream into 2 cups of the mushroom soup
just before serving. Ladle ½ cup of the soup over each serving of meatballs
and noodles. Garnish with the parsley. Serve immediately.

VARIATION **Stroganoff Over Smashed Cauliflower:** Prepare the Roasted Garlic
Smashed Cauliflower (page 74). Nest the meatballs in the cauliflower mash and
spoon the soup over the top.

PER SERVING Calories: 910; Total fat: 63g; Total carbs: 57g; Sugar: 8g; Protein: 31g; Fiber: 6g;
Sodium: 812mg

SERVES 6

Prep time: 15 minutes

Cook time: 45 minutes

POT

4 pounds bone-in beef short ribs

3 celery stalks

½ cup diced onion

3 garlic cloves, minced

1 tablespoon rice vinegar

1 tablespoon dried cilantro

½ tablespoon ground cumin

1 teaspoon minced fresh ginger

1 teaspoon dried thyme

½ teaspoon ground cardamom

½ teaspoon ground cinnamon

½ teaspoon salt

1 cup water

Pressure Cooker Spiced Short Ribs

Dairy-free · ***Egg-free*** Short ribs are an occasional indulgence at my house. This recipe is inspired by an Indian-African fusion restaurant dish that my family could not stop raving about. The spice combination, gentle flavor from celery and onion, and richness of the ribs come together to create an enticing main dish worthy of any special occasion.

1. Select the Brown/Sauté setting if using an electric pressure cooker, or warm your stove-top pressure cooker over medium-high heat. Add the short ribs and brown them on all sides.

2. To the pressure cooker pot, add all of the remaining ingredients in order.

3. Lock the lid into place. Cook at high pressure for 45 minutes. After cooking, let the pressure release naturally for 10 minutes, then quick release any remaining pressure. Unlock and remove the lid.

4. Remove and discard the celery. Use a slotted spoon or spatula to remove the short ribs. Discard the remaining liquid (or see variation 2 to make gravy). Serve immediately.

VARIATION 1 **Slow Cooker Spiced Short Ribs:** Brown the short ribs in a large skillet on the stove top, then transfer to a 6-quart slow cooker. Add the remaining ingredients, using just ½ cup of water. Cover and cook on high for 5 hours or on low for 8 hours.

VARIATION 2 **Short Ribs with Gravy:** After cooking, place 1 cup of the liquid in a small saucepan and whisk in 1 tablespoon of cornstarch. Warm just until the mixture boils, then remove from heat. Season with additional salt as needed. Ladle over the short ribs to serve.

PER SERVING Calories: 380; Total fat: 23g; Total carbs: 3g; Sugar: 1g; Protein: 38g; Fiber: 1g; Sodium: 348mg

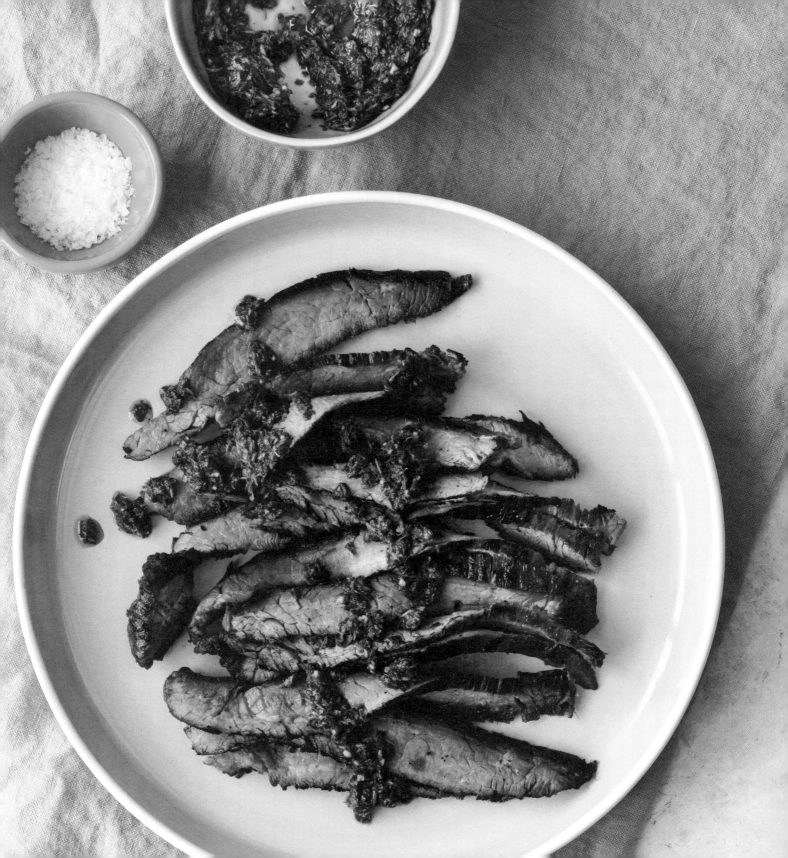

Prep time: 10 minutes,
plus 4 hours to marinate

Cook time: 15 minutes

2 tablespoons
sunflower oil

2 tablespoons freshly
squeezed lemon juice

4 garlic cloves, peeled
and halved

½ teaspoon ancho
chile powder

½ teaspoon salt

1½ pounds flank steak

Easy Flank Steak

Dairy-free · ***Egg-free*** Flank steak is an affordable cut of beef that, when prepared and cut properly, is tender and tasty. Sliced very thin, this makes great steak sandwiches, wraps, and tacos. I like to marinate the steak overnight. You can get by with less time if you need to, but 4 hours is the minimum I recommend.

1. In a small bowl, make a marinade by whisking together the oil, lemon juice, garlic, ancho chile powder, and salt.

2. Place the steak in a large, shallow baking dish. Pour the marinade over the meat and turn it to coat both sides. Cover with plastic wrap and refrigerate for at least 4 hours or up to 24 hours.

3. Set the top rack in the oven 4 to 5 inches away from the broiler. Preheat the broiler.

4. Remove the steak from the marinade and place it in a large baking pan. Discard the marinade.

5. Broil the meat, about 7 minutes per side. Test for doneness with a meat thermometer. Flank steak has the best texture when cooked to medium, about 140°F.

6. When the meat is done, remove it from the oven and let it rest for 10 minutes before transferring to a cutting board. Slice the steak very thinly against the grain, and serve.

VARIATION 1 **Curry Flank Steak:** Use 1 teaspoon of curry powder in place of the chili powder.

VARIATION 2 **Chimichurri Flank Steak:** Double the chimichurri recipe on page 89 and use half as the marinade for the meat. Save the remaining half to serve with the meat at the table.

PER SERVING Calories: 216; Total fat: 12g; Total carbs: 1g; Sugar: 0g; Protein: 25g; Fiber: 0g; Sodium: 262mg

Prep time: 10 minutes

Cook time: 8 hours

1 (1½-pound) grass-fed beef chuck roast

½ cup no-sodium chicken broth

¼ cup coconut aminos or gluten-free soy sauce

¼ cup natural apple butter

2 garlic cloves, minced

½ tablespoon sesame oil

½ tablespoon apple cider vinegar

1 teaspoon grated fresh ginger

1 teaspoon dried harissa seasoning

½ teaspoon onion powder

⅛ teaspoon freshly ground white pepper

1½ tablespoons cornstarch

Sesame seeds, for garnish (optional)

Sliced scallions, for garnish (optional)

Slow Cooker Korean Beef Roast

Dairy-free · Egg-free This roast is ultra-tender and pulls apart with a fork. I shred it and serve it with the sauce along with steamed cabbage and rice or cauliflower "rice." If you want to cut the cook time in half, cook it for 4 hours on high.

1. Place the beef roast in a 6-quart slow cooker and turn it on low heat.

2. In a small bowl, whisk together the broth, aminos, apple butter, garlic, sesame oil, vinegar, ginger, harissa, onion powder, and white pepper. Pour this over the beef.

3. Cover and cook on low for 8 hours.

4. When the beef is done, ladle about 1 cup of the liquid from the slow cooker into a small saucepan. Whisk in the cornstarch and bring to a boil. Remove from heat.

5. Carefully transfer the roast to a serving platter. Garnish with the sesame seeds and scallions (if using). Serve with the sauce.

VARIATION **Traditional Pot Roast:** Omit the aminos, apple butter, sesame oil, vinegar, ginger, harissa, onion powder, and sesame seeds. Add 6 large peeled and trimmed carrots, 1 large onion cut into 6 wedges, 6 quartered red potatoes, and ½ teaspoon of dried ground sage.

INGREDIENT TIP *If you do not have harissa seasoning, use ¼ teaspoon of garlic powder, ¼ teaspoon of ground cumin, ½ teaspoon of caraway seeds, a pinch of ground cinnamon, and ½ teaspoon of red pepper flakes.*

PER SERVING Calories: 316; Total fat: 16g; Total carbs: 5g; Sugar: 0g; Protein: 35g; Fiber: 0g; Sodium: 211mg

Apricot & Mustard–Glazed Ham

SERVES 12

Prep time: 15 minutes

Cook time: 2 to 2½ hours

5
ING

1 (10-pound) fully cooked ham, bone-in and preservative-free

1 cup all-fruit apricot jam

½ cup yellow mustard

½ teaspoon garlic powder

Dairy-free · *Egg-free* Growing up in the South, ham was served both at Easter and as an alternative to turkey at Thanksgiving. It's easy to prepare and perfect for feeding a crowd, and the leftovers are always welcome. Choose an all-natural ham, look for "gluten-free" on the label, and discard the seasoning/glaze packet if one is attached.

1. Preheat the oven to 325°F.

2. Unwrap the ham and place it in a roasting pan. Score the outer fat with a sharp knife and wrap the ham securely with aluminum foil. Bake for 1 hour.

3. While the ham is baking, make the glaze. In a small bowl, stir together the jam, mustard, and garlic powder. Reserve ⅓ cup of the mixture for serving.

4. Remove the ham from the oven and discard the foil. Baste the ham with the pan juices and half of the unreserved glaze. Return the ham to the oven and bake for 30 minutes, then baste again with the rest of the unreserved glaze. Bake the ham 30 minutes more.

5. Let the ham rest for 15 minutes before slicing.

6. While the ham rests, in a small saucepan, gently heat the ⅓ cup of reserved glaze. Serve it alongside the sliced ham.

VARIATION **Pineapple Ham:** Score the ham as directed. Place 1 whole clove in each score. In place of the apricot and mustard glaze, whisk together the juice from a 20-ounce can of pineapple rings (reserve the rings), ½ cup of brown sugar, and 2 tablespoons of yellow mustard in a small bowl. Cover the ham with the pineapple rings and place 1 stemmed maraschino cherry in the center of each ring (secure with toothpicks). Pour the pineapple glaze over the ham and bake for 2 to 2½ hours. Remove the toothpicks before slicing.

ALLERGEN TIP *If you are allergic to mustard (or do not want to use it), omit it. Ham is delicious glazed with only all-fruit jam, if you prefer. For a pop of tartness, add 1 tablespoon of fresh lemon juice to the jam.*

PER SERVING Calories: 428; Total fat: 27g; Total carbs: 9g; Sugar: 7g; Protein: 24g; Fiber: 0g; Sodium: 1567mg

1 teaspoon salt

1 teaspoon garlic powder

1 teaspoon
onion powder

1 teaspoon
smoked paprika

½ teaspoon freshly
ground black pepper

1 (3-pound) boneless
pork shoulder roast

1 small onion, peeled
and halved

1 small apple, cored
and halved

¼ cup apple
cider vinegar

1¼ cups All-American
Barbecue Sauce
(page 32), divided

¼ cup red pepper jelly

Slow Cooker Barbecue Pork

Egg-free Pork shoulder, sometimes called Boston butt, is the prime choice for pulled barbecue. It has plenty of fat to ensure moist, tender results and holds up well to vinegar-based or spicy sauces. Allow for ½ pound of boneless shoulder per person. The ingredient list seems a bit long, but the results are well worth the measuring, rubbing, and saucing involved.

1. In a small bowl, combine the salt, garlic powder, onion powder, paprika, and pepper. Rub this into the roast, coating all sides.

2. Place the roast in a 6-quart slow cooker, fattiest-side up. Add the onion, apple, vinegar, ¼ cup of barbecue sauce, and the pepper jelly.

3. Cover and cook on low for 8 hours.

4. The meat should be fork tender and easy to pull apart when it is done. Carefully transfer the roast to a large cutting board or shallow dish, and use 2 forks to pull the meat apart.

5. In a small bowl, mix together ½ cup of the cooking liquid (discard the rest) and the remaining 1 cup of barbecue sauce. Toss the meat in the sauce or serve the sauce on the side.

VARIATION **Cuban-Style Pulled Pork:** Omit the paprika, apple, vinegar, barbecue sauce, and pepper jelly. Add ½ cup of freshly squeezed orange juice and the juice of 1 lime. Chop the onion and add 4 minced garlic cloves and 2 teaspoons of ground cumin.

SUBSTITUTION TIP *Use any seasonings you like on your barbecue. If you have a favorite gluten-free barbecue rub, use 1 tablespoon of it to rub the roast before cooking. For the liquid ingredients, you can use all barbecue sauce, if you prefer.*

PER SERVING Calories: 748; Total fat: 47g; Total carbs: 41g; Sugar: 32g; Protein: 39g; Fiber: 4g; Sodium: 706mg

Prep time: 10 minutes

Cook time: 20 minutes

¼ teaspoon avocado oil or coconut oil (optional, for greasing)

1 pound ground pork

1 cup peeled and grated sweet potato

2 garlic cloves, minced

½ teaspoon dried thyme

½ teaspoon dried sage

½ teaspoon smoked paprika

½ teaspoon red pepper flakes

½ teaspoon salt

¼ teaspoon onion powder

Sweet Potato Sausage Balls

Dairy-free* · *Egg-free I created these as a grain-free alternative to traditional sausage balls that contain baking mix and cheese. They are a huge hit as an appetizer, but my family loves them for dinner, too. I double the recipe and freeze it (see the make-ahead tip), so I always have some on hand.

1. Preheat the oven to 350°F. Line a baking sheet with aluminum foil or lightly grease it with the oil.

2. In a large bowl, combine the pork, sweet potato, garlic, thyme, sage, paprika, red pepper flakes, salt, and onion powder; mix until uniform. Shape the mixture into 24 meatballs of equal size and place them on the baking sheet.

3. Bake for 20 minutes, or until cooked through.

VARIATION **Chicken Meatballs:** Substitute 1 pound of ground chicken breast for the pork, add 2 tablespoons of sunflower oil (or the meatballs will be dry), and use tarragon instead of sage; omit the red pepper flakes. Bake as directed, checking the meatballs after 15 minutes so they don't overcook.

MAKE-AHEAD TIP *Prepare through step 2. Place the sausage balls on a wax paper–lined baking sheet, and freeze until solid. Transfer to a large zip-top freezer bag or airtight freezer container. Freeze for up to 2 months. Thaw at room temperature and bake as directed.*

PER SERVING Calories: 280; Total fat: 16g; Total carbs: 11g; Sugar: 3g; Protein: 21g; Fiber: 3g; Sodium: 389mg

Prep time: 20 minutes

Cook time: 45 minutes

1 tablespoon avocado oil or coconut oil, plus ¼ teaspoon

2 (8-ounce) bone-in loin chops, about 1 inch thick

½ teaspoon salt

1 teaspoon ground cumin, divided

½ cup cooked white or brown rice

¼ cup plain Greek yogurt or dairy-free yogurt

¼ cup chopped roasted red pepper

4 tablespoons chopped fresh cilantro, divided

2 tablespoons finely chopped onion

2 tablespoons chopped fresh mint

1 garlic clove, minced

1 teaspoon gluten-free sriracha

Stuffed Pork Chops with Cumin & Fresh Herbs

Dairy-free · *Egg-free* Not everyone in my family is a pork chop fan, so I cut an old favorite recipe down to two servings. Bone-in chops are the best to use; they'll be more tender. You want them to be a bit heavy to account for the bone, so I use 8-ounce chops.

1. Preheat the oven to 350°F. Lightly grease a 9-by-9-inch baking dish with ¼ teaspoon of oil.

2. Using a sharp knife, cut into each chop opposite the bone, creating a pocket for the stuffing. Season the chops inside and out with the salt and ½ teaspoon of cumin.

3. In a small mixing bowl, stir together the rice, yogurt, red pepper, 2 tablespoons of cilantro, the onion, mint, garlic, and sriracha.

4. Divide the mixture evenly between the 2 chops, stuffing it into the pockets. Place the chops in the prepared baking dish and sprinkle with the remaining ½ teaspoon of cumin and drizzle with the remaining oil.

5. Bake for 35 to 45 minutes, until a meat thermometer inserted into the thickest part of the meat reads at least 160°F.

6. Serve hot, garnished with the remaining 2 tablespoons of cilantro.

VARIATION **Oven-Fried Pork Chops:** Omit all the ingredients except the chops, which should be a little thinner, about ½ inch thick. Preheat the oven to 450°F and grease a baking sheet with 1 tablespoon of coconut oil. Rinse the chops and pat dry with paper towels. Whisk 1 large egg in a shallow bowl. In a separate shallow bowl, whisk together 1 cup of Quick Baking Mix (page 26), 2 tablespoons of Italian seasoning, and ½ teaspoon of salt. Dip each chop in the egg, then transfer to the dry coating, turning to coat evenly. Place the chops on the baking pan. Bake for 10 minutes, then flip and bake for 10 minutes more, or until the internal temperature is 145°F.

INGREDIENT TIP *Sriracha is a spicy red chile garlic sauce. Huy Fong brand reports that their sriracha is gluten-free. Other brands are available, too.*

PER SERVING Calories: 66; Total fat: 3g; Total carbs: 9g; Sugar: 0g; Protein: 14g; Fiber: 0g; Sodium: 204mg

CHAPTER 12

Crackers, Rolls & Breads

Gluten-free baking is often easier than baking with gluten-containing flour because there's no worry about overworking the gluten and making the bread tough. Further, with gluten-free yeast breads, there is no punch down and second rise to worry about. Once you have recipes that work, like these, it's easy to bake your own bread, rolls, and crackers.

Some breads require the addition of gum to get a traditional texture. I choose guar gum and use much less than you will find in other recipes. A little really does go a long way. Ingredients and their amounts are very important in bread recipes. Pan type, pan size, and ingredient recommendations should be carefully followed to obtain the desired results.

Always ensure your gluten-free breads cool to room temperature before digging in. It's tempting to slice off a piece of fresh bread, but if you do, you may be disappointed with the texture.

Prep time: 15 minutes

Cook time: 20 minutes

150 grams (about 1 cup)
Gigi's Everyday Gluten-
Free Flour (page 27)

1 teaspoon guar gum

1 teaspoon
baking powder

½ teaspoon salt

3 tablespoons
sunflower oil

7 tablespoons water

2 teaspoons toasted
fennel seeds

1 teaspoon coarse
sea salt

Salted Fennel Crackers

Vegan This is the easiest recipe for making your own crackers. The cracker dough is mixed in the food processor and rolled out onto a large piece of parchment paper. Cut the dough right on the parchment and transfer it to the baking sheet. Couldn't get any easier! The secret to crisp-tender crackers is to roll the dough as thin as possible.

1. Preheat the oven to 375°F. Have a large (15-by-11-inch) sheet pan handy. Cut a piece of parchment paper to a size that covers it.

2. In the bowl of your food processor, place the flour, guar gum, baking powder, and salt. Pulse several times to blend. With the processor running, drizzle in the oil through the feeder opening, a little at a time. The mixture will begin to appear slightly crumb-like.

3. With the processor still running, pour in the water through the feeder opening, a little at a time, until a ball of smooth dough forms. As soon as this happens, turn off the processor. Let the dough rest in the processor while you prepare a large work area for rolling the dough.

4. Place the parchment paper on a flat surface and turn the dough out onto it. Top the dough with another piece of parchment to prevent the dough from sticking to your rolling pin.

5. Roll out the dough as thin as possible on the parchment—the thinner the better for crispiness. I roll my dough about 1/16 inch thick, about the same thickness as a U.S. penny. Once the dough is rolled out, use a sharp knife or a pizza cutter to trim the edges so it will fit on the sheet pan. Reserve the dough scraps to reroll.

6. Cut the crackers to your desired shape. I like 1½-by-1-inch rectangles. Do not separate the crackers after cutting.

7. Carefully transfer the entire sheet of parchment with the dough to a large baking sheet. Sprinkle the fennel seeds and salt over the dough. Use a fork to prick the surface of the dough, if desired.

8. Bake for approximately 20 minutes, until the crackers are golden brown. Baking time depends on thickness of the dough, so if you rolled your crackers thicker, you may need to increase the baking time.

9. Remove the baking sheet from the oven and let the crackers cool on the pan for 5 minutes.

10. Carefully transfer the crackers to a wire rack. Don't worry about breaking the crackers apart; they will easily separate when cooled. Cool them completely, then break them apart and serve.

11. Store the completely cooled crackers in an airtight container at room temperature for up to 1 week.

VARIATION 1 **Sesame Crackers:** Substitute sesame seeds for the fennel seeds and omit the coarse salt on top.

VARIATION 2 **Everything Bagel Crackers:** Omit the salt and sprinkle the crackers with "everything bagel" seasoning before baking. The "Everything but the Bagel Seasoning" from Trader Joe's is gluten-free.

INGREDIENT TIP *You may substitute another type of neutral oil for the sunflower oil, but I do not recommend olive oil in this recipe. It lends a bitter taste to the crackers.*

PER SERVING (5 crackers): Calories: 105; Total fat: 3g; Total carbs: 17g; Sugar: 1g; Protein: 1g; Fiber: 3g; Sodium: 372mg

¼ teaspoon coconut oil or avocado oil

320 grams (about 2 cups) Quick Baking Mix (page 26)

¼ teaspoon garlic powder

¼ teaspoon onion powder

2½ tablespoons mayonnaise

2 large eggs

¾ cup unsweetened coconut milk

2 teaspoons apple cider vinegar

Yeast-Free Muffin Pan Dinner Rolls

Dairy-free • ***Vegetarian*** This recipe is a huge hit with everyone who tries it. I keep the mayonnaise a secret until after folks try it, because it seems like an odd ingredient to most people. But mayo is made of eggs and oil, so it helps make these rolls tender and moist.

1. Preheat the oven to 375°F. Lightly grease a 12-cup muffin pan with the oil.

2. In a large bowl, whisk together the baking mix, garlic powder, and onion powder. Add the mayonnaise, eggs, coconut milk, and vinegar, and whisk until the batter is smooth.

3. Divide the batter evenly between the muffin cups. Bake for about 20 minutes, or until the tops rise and the centers spring back when gently pressed.

4. Cool slightly before removing from the pan and serving.

VARIATION **Herbed Rolls:** Add 2 teaspoons of dried herbs of your choice to the batter. Rosemary, thyme, and Italian seasoning are delicious in these rolls.

INGREDIENT TIP *You may omit the garlic powder and onion powder if you choose. The rolls will have a blander flavor, but it will not affect the texture of the rolls.*

PER SERVING (1 roll): Calories: 143; Total fat: 6g; Total carbs: 20g; Sugar: 1g; Protein: 3g; Fiber: 3g; Sodium: 106mg

Prep time: 5 minutes

Cook time: 15 minutes

¼ teaspoon coconut oil or avocado oil

⅔ cup milk

⅓ cup sunflower oil

1 large egg

½ teaspoon salt

165 grams (about 1½ cups) tapioca flour

½ cup finely shredded cheese, such as Cheddar, Monterey Jack, Colby, or Swiss

Easy Brazilian Rolls

Vegetarian These rolls are sometimes called Brazilian Cheese Bread. They are pleasantly gooey inside, with an exterior akin to cream puff shells. Use your blender to do all the work, or use an immersion blender for even less cleanup. Either way, you'll be rewarded with warm, cheesy rolls that pair perfectly with Creamy Tomato Soup (page 103).

1. Preheat the oven to 400°F. Grease a 24-cup mini muffin pan with the coconut or avocado oil. If you only have a 12-cup pan, bake the rolls in 2 batches and wash the pan in between.

2. In a blender, combine the milk, sunflower oil, egg, salt, and flour. Blend until smooth. Alternatively, use an immersion blender, or even a food processor if it has a snug-fitting lid, as the batter is very thin.

3. Fill the muffin cups about two-thirds full with the batter. Top each with about 1 teaspoon of the cheese.

4. Bake for 15 minutes. Serve hot. You may need to loosen the bread carefully from around the edges of the pan if some of the cheese sticks.

VARIATION **Extra-Cheesy Rolls:** Prepare as directed, but omit the salt. Sprinkle 1 teaspoon of finely grated Parmesan cheese on top of the shredded cheese for each roll. Bake as directed.

ALLERGEN TIP *To make Dairy-Free Cheesy Rolls, use dairy-free milk and dairy-free cheese. I use Daiya Cheddar shreds, and they work well.*

PER SERVING (4 rolls): Calories: 197; Total fat: 17g; Total carbs: 8g; Sugar: 1g; Protein: 4g; Fiber: 0g; Sodium: 277mg

Prep time: 5 minutes

Cook time: 15 minutes

¼ teaspoon coconut oil or avocado oil (optional, for greasing)

1 cup full-fat sour cream

¼ teaspoon guar gum

104 grams (about ¾ cup) Gigi's Everyday Gluten-Free Flour (page 27)

2 teaspoons baking powder

½ teaspoon salt

1 tablespoon melted butter

Sour Cream Dinner Rolls

Egg-free · *Vegetarian* These rolls pair well with any meal. My favorite use is as slider buns for mini burgers (see variation 2). This recipe also doubles easily, and the baked rolls freeze well for up to 2 weeks. Remember: Cooling gluten-free bread is essential to achieving excellent results in the finished product. Breads continue to cook via the steam trapped inside them. Cutting into them too soon can cause them to be gummy.

1. Preheat the oven to 375°F. Line a baking sheet with parchment paper or grease it lightly with the oil.

2. In a large bowl, stir together the sour cream and guar gum. Add the flour, baking powder, and salt. Stir until the batter is smooth. The batter will be relatively thick.

3. Spoon about 1½-tablespoon mounds of batter 2 inches apart on the baking sheet. I use a #40 cookie scoop, but a measuring spoon works just as well.

4. Brush the top of each dough mound with the melted butter, taking care not to flatten the mounds.

5. Bake for 13 to 14 minutes, or until cooked through. The bottoms will become lightly golden but the tops will not brown.

6. Let the rolls cool for at least 10 minutes before serving.

VARIATION 1 **Salted Herb Rolls:** Add up to 2 tablespoons of your favorite dried herbs to the batter, and finish with a pinch of coarse sea salt after brushing with melted butter. Dried herbs like chives, rosemary, thyme, and tarragon all work well.

VARIATION 2 **Slider Buns:** Use 2 full tablespoons of batter for each roll. After brushing the tops with melted butter, sprinkle each roll with a pinch of sesame seeds and bake as directed. Cool completely, then slice each roll in half to use as a bun. The recipe makes 10 slider buns.

PER SERVING (1 roll): Calories: 80; Total fat: 5g; Total carbs: 8g; Sugar: 0g; Protein: 1g; Fiber: 1g; Sodium: 140mg

SERVES 6

Prep time: 5 minutes

Cook time: 18 minutes

30
MIN

¼ teaspoon coconut oil or avocado oil

1 cup gluten-free cornmeal

155 grams (about 1 cup) Gigi's Everyday Gluten-Free Flour (page 27)

2 tablespoons granulated sugar

1 tablespoon baking powder

1 teaspoon salt

1 cup milk or unsweetened coconut milk

2 large eggs

⅓ cup sunflower oil

Cornbread

Dairy-free* · *Vegetarian The most popular recipe on my website has always been my cornbread recipe. It's no wonder, since cornbread is easy to make, bakes quickly, and pairs so well with soups and stews. This version is improved and streamlined and tastes delicious right out of the pan. Leftovers make delicious croutons for Southern-Style Panzanella (page 95), too!

1. Preheat the oven to 425°F. Lightly grease a 9-inch square baking pan with the coconut or avocado oil.

2. In a large bowl, combine the cornmeal, flour, sugar, baking powder, and salt. Whisk to blend. Add the milk, eggs, and sunflower oil. Whisk until the batter is smooth and no lumps are visible.

3. Pour the batter into the prepared baking pan. Bake for 25 to 30 minutes, until golden on top and crisp at the edges. Cool for 10 minutes before slicing.

VARIATION Corn Muffins with Jalapeño and Cheddar: Grease a muffin pan or line it with parchment paper liners. The recipe makes 16 muffins. Add 1 tablespoon minced jalapeño pepper, 1 cup shredded sharp Cheddar cheese, and 3 tablespoons sliced scallion to the cornbread batter. Divide the batter evenly between the muffin cups, and bake at 400°F for 15 to 18 minutes, until the tops are golden and the muffins spring back when gently pressed in center. Cool 10 minutes in the pan before serving.

ALLERGEN TIP *For egg-free cornbread, substitute prepared powdered egg replacer for the 2 eggs. I tested with Ener-G brand.*

PER SERVING Calories: 154; Total fat: 8g; Total carbs: 17g; Sugar: 3g; Protein: 4g; Fiber: 2g; Sodium: 240mg

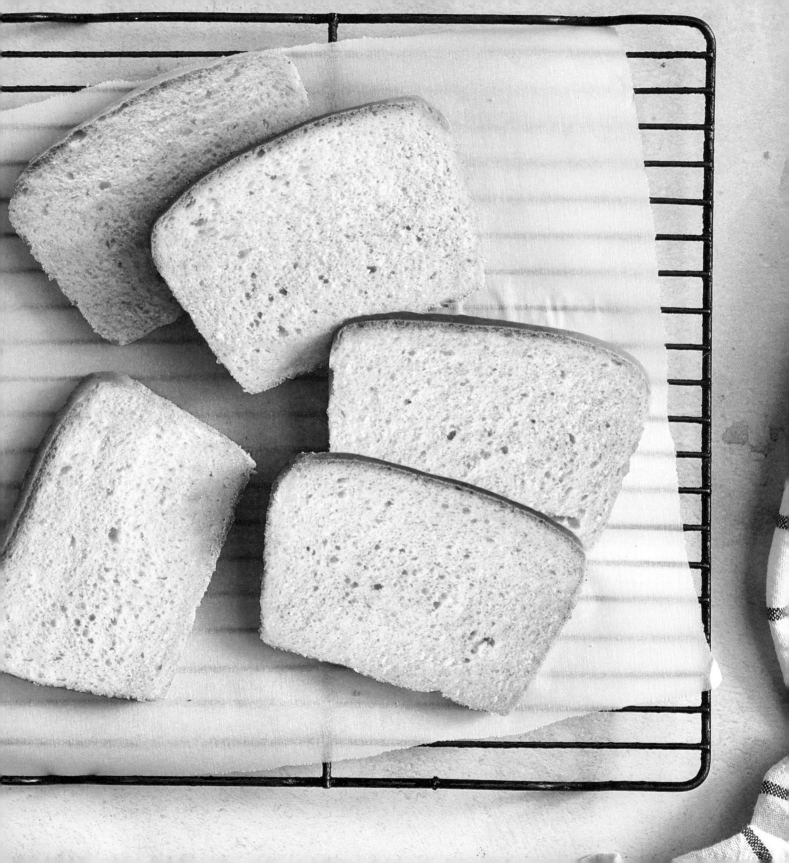

Prep time: 10 minutes,
plus 25 minutes to rise

Cook time: 50 minutes

¼ teaspoon coconut oil
or avocado oil

470 grams (about 4 cups)
Gigi's Everyday Gluten-
Free Flour (page 27)

14 grams
(2 tablespoons) sugar

6 grams (3 teaspoons)
guar gum

10 grams (2½ teaspoons)
active dry yeast

1¼ teaspoons salt

4 grams (1 teaspoon)
baking powder

1 cup water

1 cup unsweetened
coconut milk

2 tablespoons
sunflower oil

1 teaspoon apple
cider vinegar

½ tablespoon dairy-free
butter (optional)

Top 8–Free Sandwich Bread

Vegan Welcome back, delicious homemade bread! Free from
the top 8 allergens—milk, eggs, fish, crustacean shellfish, tree
nuts, peanuts, wheat, and soybeans—this bread is easy to make,
even for bread-baking newcomers. The secrets to success for this
recipe are (1) using the proper pan, (2) not allowing the bread to rise
over the top edge of the pan, and (3) cooling the bread completely
before slicing to ensure that the center will not be gummy.

1. Preheat the oven to 375°F. Lightly grease a metal 8½-by-4½-inch loaf pan
with the coconut or avocado oil.

2. Place the flour, sugar, guar gum, yeast, salt, and baking powder in the bowl
of a stand mixer. Mix briefly on low speed to blend.

3. In a medium saucepan or microwave-safe bowl, combine the water, coconut milk, and sunflower oil. Heat to 108°F, then add the apple cider vinegar.
Pour this into the dry ingredients.

4. Beat on medium speed until mixed well. Turn off the mixer, scrape down
the sides of the bowl, and mix again for about 2 minutes.

5. Spoon the batter into the loaf pan. Cover with a clean, damp kitchen towel
and set aside to rise for 25 minutes. I let my bread rise on the front edge of my
preheating oven with the door slightly ajar. If you do this, turn the pan halfway
through the rising time so one side doesn't get too hot.

6. Brush the top of the dough with melted butter (if using). This is not necessary, but the top will remain pale if you do not brush it with butter.

7. Bake for 40 to 50 minutes, or until the bread looks done on top and the internal temperature is between 190°F and 220°F.

8. Let the bread cool completely in the pan before slicing.

9. Slice and store at room temperature for 2 or 3 days, or individually wrap the slices in plastic wrap and freeze for up to 1 month.

VARIATION **Sandwich Bread with Dairy:** If you eat dairy products, use equal amounts of dairy milk and butter for the coconut milk and dairy-free butter.

SUBSTITUTION TIP *Be careful when substituting ingredients for this recipe. Yeast breads are not as agreeable to ingredient swaps as other gluten-free baked goods. Although you can substitute white vinegar for the apple cider vinegar or olive oil for the sunflower oil without issue, substituting xanthan gum for the guar gum will change the outcome. The same goes for a flour blend that contains gum. It is always best to make a recipe as written first, then make your desired adjustments, one ingredient at a time, in subsequent tries.*

PER SERVING (2 slices): Calories: 326; Total fat: 12g; Total carbs: 54g; Sugar: 6g; Protein: 5g; Fiber: 7g; Sodium: 980mg

MAKES 12 MUFFINS

Prep time: 5 minutes

Cook time: 15 minutes

¼ tablespoon coconut oil or avocado oil (optional, for greasing)

225 grams (about 1½ cups) Gigi's Everyday Gluten-Free Flour (page 27)

4 teaspoons baking powder

1 tablespoon dried chives

¼ teaspoon salt

¼ teaspoon garlic powder

¾ cup milk

2 large eggs

2 tablespoons sunflower oil

2 teaspoons honey

2 teaspoons apple cider vinegar

1 cup shredded Cheddar cheese

Cheddar & Chive Muffins

Vegetarian These savory muffins are delicious with a bowl of soup for dinner, but I also like to serve them for weekend brunch. The flavor pairs well with Perfect Scrambled Eggs (page 50), and they also make a great "bun" for crispy bacon or baked ham.

1. Preheat the oven to 375°F. Line a 12-cup muffin pan with parchment liners, or lightly grease them with the coconut or avocado oil.

2. In a large bowl, whisk together the flour, baking powder, chives, salt, and garlic powder. Add the milk, eggs, oil, honey, and vinegar. Stir until no dry ingredients remain visible. Stir in the cheese.

3. Divide the batter evenly between the muffin cups.

4. Bake for 15 minutes. Let cool for 10 minutes in the pan before serving.

VARIATION **Sun-Dried Tomato–Parmesan Muffins:** Omit the salt and Cheddar. Add ¼ cup of chopped sun-dried tomatoes, ½ cup of shredded mozzarella cheese, and ½ cup of grated Parmesan.

ALLERGEN TIP *Make the muffins dairy-free by using dairy-free milk and cheese.*

PER SERVING (1 muffin): Calories: 136; Total fat: 7g; Total carbs: 14g; Sugar: 2g; Protein: 5g; Fiber: 2g; Sodium: 129mg

300 grams (about 2 cups) Gigi's Everyday Gluten-Free Flour (page 27)

2 teaspoons fast-acting yeast

1 teaspoon sugar

¾ teaspoon salt

½ teaspoon baking soda

½ cup water

¼ cup dairy-free plain yogurt

1 tablespoon sunflower oil

1 large egg

Versatile Flatbread

Dairy-free • ***Vegetarian*** This flatbread is my version of Indian naan. It is soft and bendable, and makes great mini pizzas and wraps. I always make a batch to serve with Indian dishes. I use a pizza stone to bake the bread, but you can use a baking sheet, too. Just be sure to lightly grease it.

1. Preheat the oven to 500°F. Place an oven rack in the highest position in the oven and put a pizza stone on the rack to preheat.

2. Place the flour, yeast, sugar, salt, and baking soda in the bowl of your stand mixer. Mix on low speed for 30 seconds.

3. In a small microwave-safe bowl, stir together the water, yogurt, and oil. Warm to 108°F. Alternatively, place in a small saucepan and heat on the stove top. Pour the warm mixture into the dry ingredients and mix on low speed for 30 seconds.

4. Add the egg to the dough and mix on low for 15 seconds, then increase to medium speed for 1 minute.

5. Cover the mixing bowl with a damp, clean kitchen towel or paper towel. Set aside for 15 minutes to rise.

6. Carefully remove the pizza stone from the oven. Scoop ⅓-cup portions of dough onto the hot stone and use an offset spatula or the back of a spoon to spread the dough portions quickly into oval shapes about ⅛ inch thick. I get 3 flatbreads on my pizza stone, so I bake in 2 batches.

7. Bake for 4 to 5 minutes, until the bread is light and golden. Repeat with the remaining dough to make 3 more flatbreads.

8. Place the bread on a plate and cover with a clean cloth to keep warm until ready to serve.

VARIATION 1 **Garlic and Ghee:** After the bread is baked, spread each with 2 teaspoons of ghee and ½ teaspoon of minced garlic.

VARIATION 2 **Cheese Naan:** After shaping the dough to bake, top with small cubes of paneer cheese.

SUBSTITUTION TIP *Use plain dairy yogurt if you eat dairy.*

PER SERVING (1 piece): Calories: 214; Total fat: 4g; Total carbs: 40g; Sugar: 3g; Protein: 5g; Fiber: 5g; Sodium: 547mg

CHAPTER 13

Cakes, Cookies & More

Gluten-free baked goods have the reputation of being dry, gritty, or dense in texture. Beginning with a recipe that works is the secret to gluten-free baking success. Made as directed, these recipes will remind you how dessert should taste. In addition to the tips and troubleshooting techniques on page 10, here are some gluten-free baking recommendations to help you along the way:

- Test your oven temperature. Temperatures can vary as much as 90 degrees, causing under- or over-baking.

- Use the correct pan size and material. Metal pans are best for high-sugar sweets like brownies, because glass dishes cause over-browning.

- Follow recipes as written, keeping in mind that gluten-free batter typically does not resemble traditional batter.

- Use room-temperature ingredients (liquids, flour blend, eggs), unless specified otherwise, to give lift to baked goods.

- Only change one ingredient at a time so you know how the change affects the recipe.

- Follow cooling time directions. Foods continue to cook when removed from the oven. Some recipes rely on this.

Prep time: 15 minutes

Cook time: 35 minutes

¼ teaspoon coconut oil
or avocado oil

1 tablespoon apple
cider vinegar

1¼ cups plus
3 tablespoons unsweet-
ened coconut milk

345 grams (about 2 cups
plus 2 tablespoons)
Gigi's Everyday Gluten-
Free Flour (page 27)

1½ teaspoons
baking powder

1½ teaspoons guar gum

1 teaspoon salt

½ teaspoon baking soda

1½ cups
granulated sugar

3 large eggs

¾ cup sunflower oil

1 tablespoon pure
vanilla extract

Best Yellow Sheet Cake

Dairy-free • *Vegetarian* A sound recipe for deliciously plush yellow cake is essential, and this one delivers. It's unique because there is no fancy mixing technique to follow. There are, however, three secrets to success for this cake: Bake it in a metal pan for proper heat distribution, follow the recipe precisely as written, and trust the rare (for me) inclusion of a small amount of guar gum.

1. Preheat the oven to 350°F. Lightly grease a 9-by-13-inch metal cake pan with the coconut or avocado oil.

2. In a large measuring cup, pour the vinegar first, then add enough coconut milk to equal 1½ cups in total. Set aside.

3. Place the flour, baking powder, guar gum, salt, baking soda, and sugar in the bowl of a stand mixer. Mix on low speed for 30 seconds. Turn off the mixer.

4. Add the eggs, sunflower oil, vinegared milk, and vanilla to the mixer. Beat on low speed for 30 seconds, then increase to medium speed and blend until the batter is smooth, 1 to 2 minutes. The batter will be thin and pourable.

5. Pour the batter into the pan.

6. Bake for 30 to 35 minutes, until the cake rises and domes slightly in the center and springs back when lightly pressed.

7. Let the cake cool completely in the pan to room temperature. Frost as desired. Cut into 18 pieces to serve.

VARIATION **Yellow Cupcakes:** This recipe makes 24 cupcakes. Use parchment cupcake liners for the best results. Bake for 20 minutes.

PER SERVING (1 piece): Calories: 265; Total fat: 16g; Total carbs: 31g; Sugar: 17g; Protein: 3g; Fiber: 2g; Sodium: 165mg

Prep time: 30 minutes, plus 8 hours to chill

Cook time: 30 minutes

1 recipe Best Yellow Sheet Cake (page 198)

16 ounces full-fat sour cream

1½ cups granulated sugar

1 (6-ounce) package frozen grated coconut, thawed, divided

16 ounces heavy (whipping) cream, very cold

2 tablespoons confectioners sugar

1 teaspoon pure vanilla extract

Sour Cream Coconut Cake

Vegetarian This Southern classic is usually made with a box mix and Cool Whip. I step it up a notch by using a homemade sheet cake and real whipped cream. Find frozen grated coconut with the frozen fruit in the grocery store. Flaked coconut will not yield the same results. Don't skimp on the refrigeration time. The sour cream mixture must have time to absorb into the cake before serving.

1. Prepare the cake according to recipe directions and cool it completely in its pan.

2. Place a stand mixer bowl and whisk attachment in the refrigerator or freezer to get them very cold.

3. While the cake cools, stir together the sour cream, granulated sugar, and all but ¼ cup of the coconut in a medium bowl. Refrigerate until ready to use.

4. When the cake is completely cool, use a sharp knife to cut the cake into 18 (2-by-3-inch) pieces. Pour the sour cream mixture over the cake and spread evenly with a spatula. It may look like too much liquid for the cake, but the cake will absorb it all. Refrigerate the cake while you make the topping.

5. Add the cold heavy cream, confectioners sugar, and vanilla to the chilled bowl of the stand mixer. Using the chilled whisk attachment, whip at high speed until peaks form and the cream develops a thick, spreadable consistency, about 5 minutes.

6. Spread the cream over the cake and sprinkle with the remaining ¼ cup of coconut. Cover and refrigerate for at least 8 hours or overnight before serving.

SUBSTITUTION TIP *Substitute a container of store-bought whipped topping for the heavy cream, confectioners sugar, and vanilla.*

PER SERVING (1 piece): Calories: 507; Total fat: 34g; Total carbs: 52g; Sugar: 34g; Protein: 4g; Fiber: 3g; Sodium: 188mg

FOR THE CAKE

¼ teaspoon coconut oil or avocado oil

1 cup hot water

44 grams (about ½ cup) unsweetened cocoa powder, sifted

245 grams (about 1¼ cups) granulated sugar

½ cup sunflower oil

2 large eggs, at room temperature

1 tablespoon pure vanilla extract

320 grams (about 2 cups) Gigi's Everyday Gluten-Free Flour (page 27)

2 teaspoons baking powder

1 teaspoon baking soda

½ teaspoon salt

One-Bowl Chocolate Cake

Dairy-free · *Vegetarian* Everyday ingredients come together in a flash and yield a delicate crumb with rich chocolate flavor. "Blooming" the cocoa powder with hot water will activate the cocoa particles and produce a more intense chocolate flavor. It works in recipes with sufficient liquid (like a cake, but not cookies) that rely on cocoa powder alone for chocolate flavor. Natural or Dutch process cocoa powder both work in this recipe.

1. Preheat the oven to 350°F. Grease a 9-by-13-inch metal cake pan with the coconut or avocado oil. Set aside.

2. In the bowl of a stand mixer, combine the hot water and cocoa. Let stand for 10 minutes.

3. In this order, add the sugar, sunflower oil, eggs, vanilla, flour, baking powder, baking soda, and salt to the bowl. Mix on low speed for 30 seconds, then increase to medium speed and mix for 1 minute. Pour the batter into the pan.

4. Bake for 25 to 30 minutes, checking it after 20 minutes, as chocolate cake is more likely to overbake. The cake is done when it rises and appears dry on top. The center of the cake will spring back when lightly pressed.

5. Let the cake cool to room temperature in the pan.

FOR THE FROSTING

340 grams (about 3 cups) confectioners sugar

44 grams (about ½ cup) unsweetened cocoa powder

¼ cup dairy-free butter, at room temperature

4 tablespoons unsweetened coconut milk

2 teaspoons pure vanilla extract

¼ teaspoon salt

6. While the cake cools, make the frosting. In the bowl of the stand mixer, combine the confectioners sugar, cocoa powder, butter, coconut milk, vanilla, and salt; beat until smooth, with no dry areas remaining.

7. Once the cake is completely cooled, spread the frosting over the top.

8. Cut into squares to serve. Tightly cover leftovers and refrigerate for up to 3 days.

VARIATION 1 **Double-Chocolate Mocha Cake:** Substitute hot black coffee for the water, add ½ cup of chocolate chips to the batter, and use ⅓ cup ghee instead of the sunflower oil. Bake, cool, and frost as directed.

VARIATION 2 **Upside-Down German Chocolate Cake:** After greasing the baking pan, layer ½ cup of flaked coconut and ½ cup of chopped pecans (or sunflower or pumpkin seeds, if you do not eat nuts) in the pan. Prepare the cake batter as directed and pour it into the pan. In a separate bowl, blend 8 ounces of cream cheese, 2 cups of confectioners sugar, and 2 tablespoons of room-temperature butter until smooth. Drop tablespoons of this on the cake batter. Bake as directed. Cool the cake completely (do not frost). Once the cake is completely cooled, turn it onto a large cake board. Slice and serve.

SUBSTITUTION TIP *For the frosting, substitute butter for the dairy-free butter and milk or cream for the coconut milk.*

PER SERVING (1 piece): Calories: 243; Total fat: 11g; Total carbs: 36g; Sugar: 20g; Protein: 3g; Fiber: 4g; Sodium: 249mg

SERVES 12

Prep time: 15 minutes

Cook time: 22 minutes

FOR THE CAKE

¼ teaspoon coconut oil or avocado oil

320 grams (about 2 cups) Gigi's Everyday Gluten-Free Flour (page 27)

1 cup coconut sugar

2 teaspoons baking soda

2 teaspoons ground cinnamon

1 teaspoon baking powder

½ teaspoon ground ginger

½ teaspoon salt

¼ teaspoon ground nutmeg

3 large eggs

1 (8-ounce) can crushed pineapple, drained; reserve the liquid

1 cup buttermilk

2 tablespoons sunflower oil

2 tablespoons melted butter

2 teaspoons pure vanilla extract

2 cups grated carrots

Carrot Cake with Cream Cheese Frosting

Vegetarian This lower-fat carrot cake is moist, flavorful, and lightly spiced. The addition of crushed pineapple adds sweetness and helps keep the cake moist. For the best texture, I grate the carrots myself; I find pre-shredded carrots to be too coarse for this cake.

1. Preheat the oven to 350°F. Lightly grease 2 (9-inch) metal cake pans with the coconut or avocado oil.

2. In the bowl of your stand mixer, combine the flour, sugar, baking soda, cinnamon, baking powder, ginger, salt, and nutmeg. Mix on low speed for 30 seconds.

3. Add the eggs, pineapple, buttermilk, sunflower oil, butter, and vanilla. Mix on low speed for 30 seconds, then increase to medium speed and mix until the batter is smooth, about 2 minutes. Fold in the carrots with a spatula.

4. Spoon the batter into the cake pans. Bake for about 22 minutes, or until the center of each cake springs back when lightly touched.

5. Spoon the reserved pineapple juice over the warm cakes. Let the cakes cool completely in the pans before removing.

FOR THE FROSTING

8 ounces cream cheese, at room temperature

450 grams (about 4 cups) confectioners sugar, divided

2 tablespoons heavy (whipping) cream

1 teaspoon pure vanilla extract

6. To make the frosting, combine the cream cheese and 2 cups of confectioners sugar in the bowl of the stand mixer. Beat until smooth.

7. Add the cream and vanilla and beat until incorporated. Add the remaining 2 cups of confectioners sugar, 1 cup at a time, beating after each addition until smooth and fluffy. If the frosting seems too thick, add a tablespoon of additional cream.

8. Remove the cooled cakes from the pans. Fill and frost the layers. Refrigerate until ready to serve.

VARIATION **Raisin-Pecan Carrot Cake:** Add ½ cup each of raisins and chopped pecans to the cake batter along with the carrots.

ALLERGEN TIP *To make a dairy-free carrot cake, put 1 tablespoon apple cider vinegar in a measuring cup. Fill to 1 cup with dairy-free milk. Use this instead of the buttermilk. For the butter, use 2 tablespoons melted dairy-free butter. Cover with the Vegan Cream Cheese Frosting (page 219).*

PER SERVING (1 slice): Calories: 359; Total fat: 14g; Total carbs: 55g; Sugar: 31g; Protein: 6g; Fiber: 4g; Sodium: 510mg

SERVES 16

Prep time: 25 minutes, plus overnight to chill

Cook time: 1 hour 20 minutes

FOR THE CRUST

¼ teaspoon coconut oil or avocado oil

2 cups gluten-free graham cracker crumbs

⅓ cup light brown sugar, firmly packed

8 tablespoons melted butter

FOR THE FILLING

5 (8-ounce) packages cream cheese, at room temperature

5 large eggs, at room temperature

1 cup granulated sugar

1 cup sour cream, at room temperature

38 grams (about ¼ cup) Gigi's Everyday Gluten-Free Flour (page 27)

1 tablespoon pure vanilla extract

New York–Style Cheesecake

Vegetarian I'm no New Yorker, but I know a good cheesecake when I taste one. Five blocks of cream cheese make this one rise to the top of the springform pan. The crust is the best graham-style crust you'll ever taste; it's more like a delicate candy than the grainy, crumbly crust usually on cheesecake. I use Kinnikinnick gluten-free graham cracker crumbs. The crust can be used for any recipe requiring a graham-style crust. Serve this recipe as-is for cheesecake bliss.

TO MAKE THE CRUST

1. Preheat the oven to 325°F. Grease a 9-inch springform pan with the oil.

2. In a medium bowl, stir together the graham crumbs and sugar. Drizzle the butter over the crumbs and stir until the crumbs are coated.

3. Transfer the crust to the springform pan. Use a flat-bottomed measuring cup to press the crust firmly and evenly into place across the bottom and ½ inch up the sides of the pan. Bake for 10 minutes. Remove from the oven, and leave the oven on.

TO MAKE THE FILLING

1. Place the cream cheese in the bowl of a stand mixer. Beat on medium speed until smooth. Add the eggs, one at a time, beating after each addition just until incorporated. Do not overbeat the eggs.

2. Add the sugar and beat just until blended.

3. Add the sour cream and beat until fully incorporated.

4. Add the flour and vanilla and beat until no dry ingredients are visible. Turn off the mixer, scrape the bottom and sides of the bowl, and then beat one final time to make sure all the ingredients are mixed well.

TO MAKE THE CHEESECAKE

1. Spoon the filling into the crust.

2. Bake for 1 hour and 10 minutes. The top of the cheesecake will appear slightly dry and less glossy, and it may crack (this is normal; steam is escaping).

3. Remove the cheesecake from the oven and let it cool completely at room temperature. Once cooled, refrigerate overnight before removing it from the pan.

4. The next day, carefully remove the pan sides and transfer the cheesecake, still on the pan base, to a serving tray. To serve, slice the cheesecake into wedges. Refrigerate leftovers in an airtight container for up to 1 week.

ALLERGEN TIP *To make the crust dairy-free, I substitute Earth Balance Soy Free Buttery Spread for the butter.*

PER SERVING Calories: 467; Total fat: 36g; Total carbs: 29g; Sugar: 18g; Protein: 9g; Fiber: 1g; Sodium: 382mg

SERVES 8

Prep time: 15 minutes

Cook time: 25 minutes

FOR THE BATTER

¼ teaspoon coconut oil or avocado oil

228 grams (about 1½ cups) Quick Baking Mix (page 26)

½ cup granulated sugar

2 large eggs

½ cup unsweetened coconut milk

2 tablespoons sunflower oil

Juice of 1 lemon

1 cup blueberries

FOR THE STREUSEL

100 grams (about ⅔ cup) Quick Baking Mix (page 26)

½ cup granulated sugar

1½ teaspoons ground cinnamon

¼ cup dairy-free butter

Zest of 1 lemon

Blueberry Coffee Cake

Dairy-free • *Vegetarian* I find coffee cake too sweet for breakfast, but I love it for dessert. This version is easy to put together with my Quick Baking Mix (page 26), which already contains the leavening. Use fresh blueberries when in season. Frozen blueberries also work, but you may need to add a few extra minutes to the baking time.

1. Preheat the oven to 350°F. Grease a 9-inch square or round baking pan with the coconut or avocado oil.

2. To make the batter, in a large bowl, stir together the baking mix, sugar, eggs, milk, sunflower oil, and lemon juice until a smooth batter forms. Gently fold in the blueberries. Pour the batter into the prepared baking pan.

3. To make the streusel, in a small bowl, combine the baking mix, sugar, cinnamon, butter, and lemon zest. Use a fork to cut in the butter. The topping should look like coarse crumbs.

4. Top the batter with the streusel, gently pressing it into the batter.

5. Bake for 20 to 25 minutes. Let cool for 20 minutes before slicing and serving.

VARIATION 1 **Chocolate Chip Coffee Cake:** Add ⅓ cup of mini chocolate chips to the batter and omit the lemon juice and blueberries. Add ⅓ cup of mini chocolate chips to the topping and omit the lemon zest.

VARIATION 2 **Coffee Cake Muffins:** Grease a 12-cup muffin tin and divide the batter evenly between the cups. Top each cup with some of the streusel, gently pressing it into the batter. Bake for 18 to 20 minutes. Let cool in the pan for 20 minutes before serving.

PER SERVING Calories: 388; Total fat: 15g; Total carbs: 62g; Sugar: 29g; Protein: 5g; Fiber: 6g; Sodium: 185mg

Prep time: 10 minutes

Cook time: 10 minutes

240 grams (about
1½ cups) Quick Baking
Mix (page 26)

¾ cup granulated sugar

2 teaspoons
ground ginger

1 teaspoon ground
cinnamon

½ teaspoon
ground nutmeg

¼ teaspoon salt

1 large egg

¼ cup palm shortening,
at room temperature

1 teaspoon pure
vanilla extract

Delicate Ginger Cookies

Dairy-free • ***Vegetarian*** These big spice cookies have a light-as-air texture and delicate flavor. Be sure to space them far enough apart on the baking sheet so they don't run together, as they will spread during baking.

1. Preheat the oven to 350°F. Line a large baking sheet with parchment paper.

2. In a large bowl, whisk together the baking mix, sugar, ginger, cinnamon, nutmeg, and salt. Add the egg, shortening, and vanilla. Stir until the batter is smooth.

3. Scoop level tablespoon measures of batter onto the baking sheet, spacing the cookies 2½ inches apart. Bake for 8 to 10 minutes. Let the cookies cool on the baking sheet for 10 minutes, then transfer them a wire rack to finish cooling.

VARIATION 1 **Chocolate Chip Spice Cookies:** Add ⅓ cup semisweet chocolate chips to the batter.

VARIATION 2 **Cinnamon Spice Cookies:** Use 2 teaspoons of ground cinnamon, ¼ teaspoon of nutmeg, and ¼ teaspoon of ground ginger in the cookies. Combine 1 tablespoon of granulated sugar and 2 teaspoons of ground cinnamon, and sprinkle over the cookies before baking.

PER SERVING (1 cookie): Calories: 84; Total fat: 3g; Total carbs: 15g; Sugar: 7g; Protein: 1g; Fiber: 1g; Sodium: 56mg

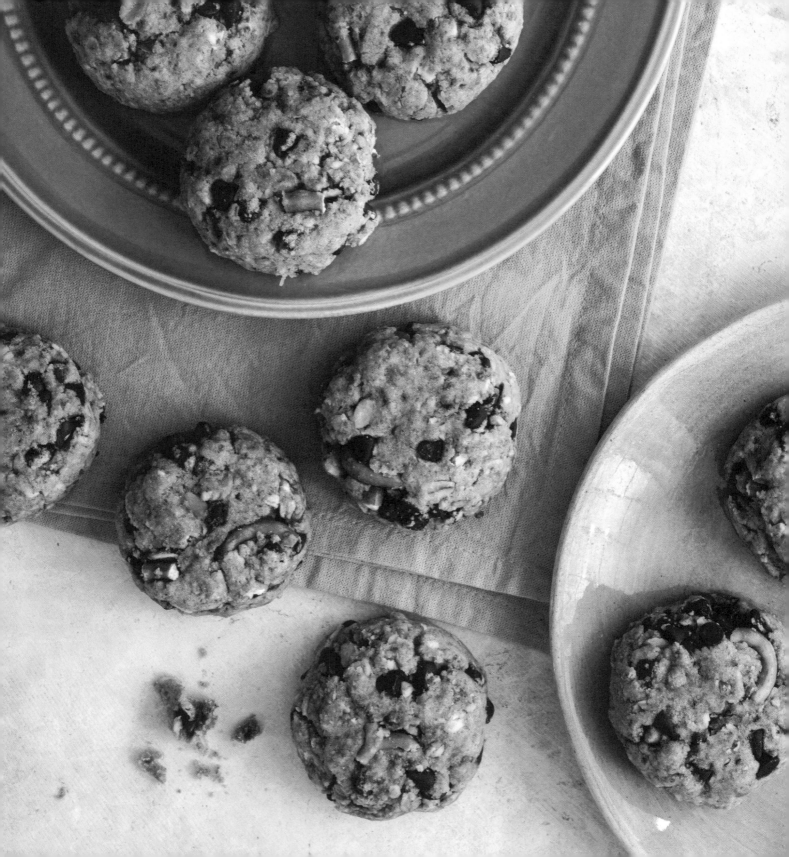

1 tablespoon
flaxseed meal

3 tablespoons
warm water

⅓ cup unsalted,
no-sugar-added
sunflower seed butter

¼ cup palm shortening,
at room temperature

½ cup coconut sugar

2 teaspoons pure
vanilla extract

¼ teaspoon salt

120 grams (about
1½ cups) purity
protocol oats

80 grams (about ½ cup)
Quick Baking Mix
(page 26)

½ cup crushed
gluten-free pretzels

½ cup vegan dark
chocolate chips

Sweet-and-Salty Chocolate Chip Cookies

Vegan If you love the combination of sweet and salty, this is your new favorite cookie. I love how crunchy the pretzels remain after baking. I use Glutino brand pretzels and vegan dark chocolate in this recipe. For a beautiful presentation, save a few pretzel pieces and chocolate chips to press into the top of each cookie before baking.

1. Preheat the oven to 350°F. Line a large baking sheet with parchment paper.

2. In a small bowl, whisk the flaxseed into the water.

3. In a large bowl, stir together the sunflower seed butter, shortening, sugar, vanilla, and salt until creamy and smooth. Stir in the flaxseed-water mixture.

4. Add the oats and baking mix and stir until no dry ingredients remain visible. Stir in the pretzels and chocolate chips.

5. Scoop 1½-tablespoon portions onto the baking sheet, spacing them a few inches apart. Gently flatten each cookie by hand. Bake for 10 minutes. Let cool on the baking sheet for 15 minutes before serving.

VARIATION **Peanut Butter White Chocolate Chip Cookies:** Substitute peanut butter for the sunflower seed butter and white chocolate chips for the chocolate. Be sure that your white chips are gluten-free.

SUBSTITUTION TIP *Substitute chia seeds for the flaxseed meal.*

PER SERVING Calories: 136; Total fat: 6g; Total carbs: 19g; Sugar: 7g; Protein: 3g; Fiber: 1g; Sodium: 150mg

Prep time: 10 minutes

Cook time: 10 minutes

30
MIN

½ cup palm shortening

85 grams (heaping ½ cup) coconut sugar

1 large egg

½ tablespoon pure vanilla extract

½ teaspoon salt

80 grams (about ½ cup) Quick Baking Mix (page 26)

½ teaspoon ground cinnamon

135 grams (about 1½ cups) purity protocol oats

½ cup dark chocolate chips

½ cup seedless Thompson or golden raisins

½ cup toasted salted pumpkin seeds

Chocolate Chip Oatmeal Cookies

Dairy-free · ***Vegetarian*** Oats are a wild-card ingredient in gluten-free baking. Not everyone with celiac disease or another gluten-related health issue can tolerate oats. I recommend gluten-free purity protocol grown oats. Shortening is also worth mentioning. Because shortening is pure fat, it prevents excessive spreading during baking. I use and recommend Nutiva organic palm shortening, which is free of trans fats.

1. Preheat the oven to 350°F. Line a baking sheet with parchment paper.

2. In a medium bowl, vigorously stir together the shortening and sugar until the shortening softens. Add the egg and stir vigorously to incorporate.

3. Add the vanilla, salt, baking mix, cinnamon, and oats. Stir just until blended. Stir in the chocolate chips, raisins, and pumpkin seeds just enough to evenly distribute them in the batter.

4. Scoop 1½-tablespoon portions of batter onto the baking sheet, spacing them a few inches apart. Gently press the top of each cookie to flatten slightly.

5. Bake for 10 minutes, then cool on the baking sheet for at least 15 minutes. The cookies need this time to firm up before you transfer them to a serving plate.

VARIATION 1 **Oatmeal Cinnamon Raisin Cookies:** Omit the chocolate chips. Increase the cinnamon to 1½ teaspoons. The pumpkin seeds are optional.

VARIATION 2 **Salted Walnut Chunk Cookies:** If you can eat nuts, substitute ½ cup of chopped walnuts for the pumpkin seeds and use chocolate chunks in place of chocolate chips. After slightly flattening the cookie dough, sprinkle each cookie with a pinch of coarse sea salt.

PER SERVING (1 cookie): Calories: 106; Total fat: 6g; Total carbs: 12g; Sugar: 7g; Protein: 1g; Fiber: 0g; Sodium: 70mg

Prep time: 15 minutes

Cook time: 45 minutes

¼ teaspoon coconut oil or avocado oil

6 cups hulled and halved strawberries

¼ cup sugar

½ cup plus 3 table-spoons Gigi's Everyday Gluten-Free Flour (page 27), divided

1 cup purity protocol oats

½ cup light brown sugar

¼ teaspoon salt

¼ cup dairy-free butter

Strawberry Crumble

Vegan You may only need 2 tablespoons of sugar for the filling, rather than the ¼ cup listed, depending on the sweetness of the strawberries. Taste the berries. If they are very sweet, like they are during peak season, use less sugar. Early or late in the season, when berries aren't as sweet and juicy, use the full amount of sugar. More sugar yields a juicier filling.

1. Preheat the oven to 350°F. Lightly grease a 9-inch glass deep-dish pie plate with the oil. Place the pie plate on a baking sheet to catch any juice that bubbles over during baking.

2. Place the strawberries in the pie plate and sprinkle with the sugar and 3 tablespoons of flour. Gently stir to combine.

3. Place the oats, brown sugar, salt, butter, and the remaining ½ cup of flour in the bowl of a food processor. Pulse until the mixture resembles coarse crumbs. Spread the topping evenly over the strawberries.

4. Bake for about 45 minutes, until the filling bubbles up along the edge of the baking dish and the topping is golden brown. Let cool for 30 minutes before serving.

VARIATION **Blueberry Crumble:** Use blueberries instead of strawberries. Add 1 tablespoon of freshly squeezed lemon juice to the berry mixture, and add the zest of 1 lemon to the topping.

ALLERGEN TIP *If you are not able to eat oats, substitute with ¾ cup of chopped nuts. Pecans are an excellent choice.*

PER SERVING Calories: 198; Total fat: 7g; Total carbs: 34g; Sugar: 20g; Protein: 3g; Fiber: 4g; Sodium: 118mg

SERVES 8

Prep time: 40 minutes

Cook time: 45 minutes

FOR THE PIE

1 recipe Pie Crust
(page 37), unbaked

3 large Granny
Smith apples

3 large Fuji apples

⅓ cup brown sugar

¼ cup Gigi's Everyday
Gluten-Free Flour
(page 27)

1 tablespoon freshly
squeezed lemon juice

2 teaspoons
ground cinnamon

½ teaspoon
ground nutmeg

Double-Crust Apple Pie

Dairy-free · ***Vegetarian*** For the best-flavored apple pie, use at least two varieties of apple. Honeycrisp, Pippin, Jonagold, Granny Smith, and Fuji are good choices for pie. Save Red Delicious apples for snacking. They are too grainy for baking into a pie.

1. Preheat the oven to 375°F.

2. Prepare the pie crust and divide the dough into 2 portions, one slightly larger than the other. Cover the smaller portion with plastic wrap and set it aside.

3. Roll the larger dough portion into a circle about 12 inches in diameter. Fit it into a 9-inch glass deep-dish pie plate. The dough will fall over the edges slightly.

4. Peel, core, and cut the apples into ¼-inch-thick slices. Place them in a large bowl and add the sugar, flour, lemon juice, cinnamon, and nutmeg. Gently stir to coat the apple slices, being careful not to break them. Spoon the apple mixture into the crust.

5. Roll out the top crust to about 9 inches in diameter. Place it over the filling in the pie plate. Take the overlapping edge of the bottom crust and roll it over the edge of the top crust, crimping to secure. Use a sharp knife to cut several slits into the top crust so that steam can escape during baking.

FOR THE SHINY TOP CRUST (OPTIONAL)

1 egg white

2 teaspoons water

½ tablespoon coarse sugar

6. *Optional step:* If you'd like to make a shiny top crust, whisk together the egg white and water in a small bowl. Lightly brush this over the top crust. You will not use all of it. Sprinkle the sugar over the crust.

7. Place the pie plate on a large baking sheet in case of filling overflow. Bake for 30 minutes, then check the crust. If it becomes too brown before the pie is done, use strips of aluminum foil to lightly cover the crust edges. Bake the pie for about another 15 minutes, until the filling is bubbling and the crust is golden brown.

8. Cool the pie completely before slicing.

VARIATION 1 **Double-Crust Fruit Pie:** Substitute about 6 cups of mixed fresh fruit for the apples.

VARIATION 2 **Single-Crust Crumb-Topped Pie:** Make the pie as directed through step 4, but save the top crust for another pie or freeze it for later use. In a food processor, pulse together ½ cup of Gigi's Everyday Gluten-Free Flour, ½ cup of sugar, ¼ cup of dairy-free butter, ¼ teaspoon of cinnamon, and ¼ teaspoon of salt until it resembles crumbs. Press this crumb topping into the pie filling and bake.

INGREDIENT TIP *Lemon juice keeps the apples from overbrowning during baking. If you cannot eat citrus, omit the lemon juice. Cinnamon and nutmeg are not essential to the recipe outcome, so if you cannot eat those, feel free to omit.*

PER SERVING Calories: 335; Total fat: 21g; Total carbs: 64g; Sugar: 24g; Protein: 3g; Fiber: 6g; Sodium: 94mg

Prep time: 20 minutes, plus overnight to chill

Cook time: 55 minutes

1 (9-inch) Pie Crust (page 37), unbaked

1½ cups roughly chopped toasted pumpkin seeds or sunflower seeds

1¼ cups semisweet or dark chocolate chips

2 large eggs

½ cup light brown sugar, firmly packed

½ cup granulated sugar

4 tablespoons tapioca flour

4 tablespoons dairy-free butter, melted and cooled

1 teaspoon pure vanilla extract

¼ teaspoon salt

3 tablespoons bourbon (optional)

Chocolate Kentucky Bourbon Pie

Dairy-free · Vegetarian This recipe is one I make each May as part of our Kentucky Derby celebration. It traditionally calls for walnuts in the filling, but because of a nut allergy, I use toasted pumpkin or sunflower seed kernels. Make this recipe at least one day before you plan to serve it, because it must cool completely at room temperature, then be refrigerated overnight before slicing.

1. Preheat the oven to 325°F.

2. Prepare the pie crust by rolling out the dough and fitting it into a nonmetal 9-inch pie plate.

3. Spread the seeds evenly over the bottom of the pie dough and top with the chocolate chips.

4. In the bowl of your stand mixer, beat the eggs for 1 minute at medium-high speed. Add the brown sugar, granulated sugar, flour, butter, vanilla, salt, and bourbon (if using), and beat for 45 seconds on medium speed. Pour into the dough.

5. Place the pie plate on a baking sheet. Bake for 45 to 55 minutes, until the top is dry and the edges begin to turn golden brown.

6. Let the pie cool completely to room temperature. Refrigerate overnight. The pie must be completely chilled to slice properly. Serve cold or at room temperature with vanilla ice cream or whipped cream, if desired.

VARIATION **Traditional Walnut Derby Pie:** Substitute 1½ cups of chopped walnuts or pecans for the seeds. The nuts do not need to be toasted.

PER SERVING Calories: 536; Total fat: 32g; Total carbs: 70g; Sugar: 42g; Protein: 6g; Fiber: 1g; Sodium: 184mg

Prep time: 10 minutes,
plus 2 hours to chill

NO COOK | 5 ING

½ cup Key lime juice

1 can dairy-free sweetened condensed milk

1 (9-ounce) container frozen dairy-free whipped topping, partially thawed, plus additional for garnish (optional)

½ cup gluten-free graham-style cracker crumbs, divided

Three-Ingredient Key Lime Parfait

Vegan I believe the brands matter for this recipe. I use Nellie & Joe's Key lime juice, Nature's Charm dairy-free sweetened condensed milk, So Delicious CocoWhip! topping, and Kinnikinnick graham-style crackers. The chilling time is necessary for the mixture to set up properly.

1. In a large bowl, whisk together the lime juice, sweetened condensed milk, and whipped topping until combined.

2. Divide half the mixture evenly between 4 dessert dishes. Top each with 1 tablespoon of graham crumbs. Add the remaining filling, then sprinkle another 1 tablespoon of graham crumbs on top of each serving.

3. Chill for at least 2 hours. Garnish each serving with 1 tablespoon of additional whipped topping (if using).

VARIATION **Lemon Cream Parfaits:** Substitute freshly squeezed lemon juice for the Key lime juice.

INGREDIENT TIP *If you are not dairy-free, use regular sweetened condensed milk and whipped topping.*

PER SERVING Calories: 212; Total fat: 7g; Total carbs: 32g; Sugar: 23g; Protein: 4g; Fiber: 1g; Sodium: 138mg

Prep time: 10 minutes

Cook time: 40 minutes

FOR THE CRUST

150 grams (about 1 cup) Gigi's Everyday Gluten-Free Flour (page 27)

5 tablespoons palm shortening

28 grams (about ¼ cup) confectioners sugar

FOR THE FILLING

¾ cup granulated sugar

2 large eggs

38 grams (about ¼ cup) Gigi's Everyday Gluten-Free Flour (page 27)

Zest and juice of 2 lemons

¼ teaspoon salt

Lemon Bars

Dairy-free • Vegetarian Lining the baking pan with parchment paper that overhangs two sides helps when it's time to lift out the cooled lemon bars. Place the pan on a raised wire rack to cool the bars completely to room temperature before lifting them out of the pan. A dusting of confectioners sugar is an optional finish for these bars.

1. Preheat the oven to 350°F. Line an 8-by-8-inch square metal baking pan with parchment paper that overhangs the edges of the pan.

2. To make the crust, combine the flour, shortening, and confectioners sugar in the bowl of a food processor. Pulse until the mixture resembles coarse crumbs.

3. Transfer the mixture to the baking pan and press firmly and evenly into the pan, going about ½ inch up the sides. Bake for 20 minutes. Set the crust aside to cool while you prepare the filling.

4. To make the filing, combine the sugar and eggs in the bowl of a stand mixer. Mix on low speed for 30 seconds, then increase to high speed and mix for 2 minutes. Add the flour, zest, juice, and salt, then mix for 1 minute on medium speed.

5. Pour the filling into the crust and bake for 25 to 30 minutes, until the center filling is set.

6. Place the pan on a wire rack to cool completely before removing the bars from the pan and slicing into squares.

VARIATION **Lime Bars:** Use the zest and juice of 2 limes in place of the lemon zest and juice.

INGREDIENT TIP *If you do not have a zester, use the smallest holes on a box grater to zest the lemon. Zest the lemon first, then cut it in half to extract the juice.*

PER SERVING (1 bar): Calories: 178; Total fat: 8g; Total carbs: 25g; Sugar: 13g; Protein: 3g; Fiber: 0g; Sodium: 68mg

Prep time: 10 minutes

Cook time: 25 minutes

¼ teaspoon coconut oil or avocado oil

6 ounces dairy-free butter

3 ounces 70% dark chocolate

1 cup granulated sugar

3 large eggs

2 tablespoons pure maple syrup

⅔ cup Hershey's Special Dark Dutch process cocoa

½ cup Gigi's Everyday Gluten-Free Flour (page 27)

½ teaspoon salt

Classic Brownies

Dairy-free • ***Vegetarian*** Dutch process cocoa and dark chocolate yield dark, rich brownies. For best results, use a metal baking pan, beat the eggs and sugar together for the full time indicated, and stir by hand when instructed. Do not overbake; the brownies continue to cook after they come out of the oven. Cool completely before slicing, and you'll be richly rewarded.

1. Preheat the oven to 350°F. Lightly grease an 8-by-8-inch metal baking pan with the oil.

2. In a small microwave-safe bowl, place the butter and chocolate. Microwave for 30 seconds, stirring every 10 seconds, just until the chocolate is melted. Alternatively, place the ingredients in a small saucepan over low heat and melt them together. Set aside to cool.

3. In a large bowl, use a hand mixer to beat the sugar and eggs together for 3 minutes. Add the maple syrup and stir by hand to combine.

4. In a medium bowl, sift together the cocoa powder, flour, and salt. Add this to the wet ingredients and stir by hand until no dry ingredients remain. Stir in the butter and chocolate mixture. Pour the batter into the baking pan.

5. Bake for 25 minutes. Let the brownies cool completely in the pan before slicing into squares.

PER SERVING (1 brownie): Calories: 263; Total fat: 16g; Total carbs: 30g; Sugar: 21g; Protein: 4g; Fiber: 4g; Sodium: 279mg

NO · COOK · 5 ING · 30 MIN

Heaping ½ cup Medjool dates, pitted

⅓ cup no-sugar-added sunflower seed butter

⅓ cup Hershey's Special Dark Dutch process cocoa

2 teaspoons pure vanilla extract

¼ teaspoon salt

2 tablespoons chocolate chips

Healthier No-Bake Brownies

Egg-free · *Vegetarian* These aren't brownies in the traditional sense, but they are full of rich chocolate flavor and natural sweetness from the dates. I recommend Lily's™ Dark Chocolate Premium Baking Chips, which have no added sugar. I cut the brownies into small squares and store them in the freezer so I always have a healthier treat on hand. You will need a small, ungreased glass dish or metal pan for this recipe. I use a small 8-by-5-inch glass dish, but an 8½-by-4½-inch loaf pan or any small dish will work. You can also press 1-inch balls of the mixture into the cups of a mini muffin tin for a preportioned treat.

1. In the bowl of a food processor, place the dates and sunflower seed butter. Pulse several times to break down the dates. Stop the processor and scrape down the sides of the bowl. Process until the mixture is completely smooth, scraping down the sides of the bowl again as needed, 2 to 5 minutes.

2. Add the cocoa powder, vanilla, and salt. Process until completely smooth, scraping down the sides of the bowl once or twice.

3. Spoon the mixture into an 8-by-5-inch glass dish. Place a piece of wax paper over the mixture and press down firmly with your hand, or use the flat bottom of a measuring cup to flatten and even out the "batter."

4. Remove the wax paper. Top with the chocolate chips, pressing them into the brownies a bit. Slice and serve right away, or chill until you're ready to serve. Refrigerate in an airtight container for up to 1 week or freeze for up to 1 month.

VARIATION **Peanut Butter No-Bake Brownies:** Use an equal amount of peanut butter in place of the sunflower seed butter. In fact, you can use any nut or seed butter you like in this recipe. They all work.

PER SERVING (1 brownie): Calories: 213; Total fat: 10g; Total carbs: 30g; Sugar: 22g; Protein: 5g; Fiber: 5g; Sodium: 59mg

**MAKES ABOUT
2½ CUPS**

Prep time: 15 minutes

COOK   MIN   POT

**400 grams (about
3½ cups) confectioners
sugar, divided**

½ cup palm shortening

**1½ tablespoons
unsweetened
coconut milk**

**1 tablespoon freshly
squeezed lemon juice**

**½ teaspoon
vanilla extract**

½ teaspoon rice vinegar

¼ teaspoon salt

Vegan Cream Cheese Frosting

Vegan There's no perfect match for the unique tangy flavor of cream cheese, but for those of us who must forgo dairy, this vegan version is a scrumptious substitute. This unique blend of ingredients yields the proper texture and sweet-tangy flavor that complements sweet cake layers.

1. In the bowl of a stand mixer, combine 1 cup of sugar and the shortening. Beat on low speed until smooth.

2. Add the milk, lemon juice, vanilla, vinegar, salt, and the remaining 2½ cups of sugar. Beat on low speed for 30 seconds, then increase to medium-high speed for 2 to 3 minutes, until the frosting is fluffy. You may need to scrape down the sides of your mixing bowl once or twice during mixing.

VARIATION Chocolate "Cream Cheese" Frosting: Add ½ cup of natural vegan cocoa powder and an additional 2 to 4 tablespoons of coconut milk to achieve your desired consistency.

INGREDIENT TIP *Use any dairy-free milk you like in place of coconut milk.*

PER SERVING (2 tablespoons): Calories: 135; Total fat: 6g; Total carbs: 21g; Sugar: 0g; Protein: 0g; Fiber: 0g; Sodium: 31mg

Prep time: 10 minutes

Cook time: 15 minutes

¼ teaspoon coconut oil or avocado oil

240 grams (about 1½ cups) Quick Baking Mix (page 26)

85 grams (about ½ cup) coconut sugar, plus 2 tablespoons

3 teaspoons ground cinnamon, divided

½ teaspoon ground nutmeg

½ cup unsweetened applesauce

⅓ cup unsweetened coconut milk

2 tablespoons sunflower oil

1 large egg

2 teaspoons pure vanilla extract

1 tablespoon dairy-free butter, melted

Baked Cinnamon Sugar Donuts

Dairy-free • *Vegetarian* Making donuts at home is as easy as baking muffins. You need a donut pan, but it's an inexpensive investment (about $8) considering how much use you're likely to get out of it once you taste a warm-from-the-oven cinnamon sugar donut. The addition of applesauce may sound odd, but it allows for the use of less oil without sacrificing moisture.

1. Preheat the oven to 350°F. Lightly grease a donut pan with the coconut or avocado oil. A standard donut pan makes 6 donuts, so you will need 2 rounds of baking. Wash the pan between batches.

2. In a large bowl, combine the flour, 85 grams of sugar, 1 teaspoon of cinnamon, the nutmeg, applesauce, milk, sunflower oil, egg, and vanilla. Beat by hand for 50 strokes, until no dry ingredients remain.

3. Fill a piping bag or a large zip-top plastic bag with the batter. Cut off the tip of the piping bag or a corner of the zip-top bag, and pipe the batter into the donut pan.

4. Bake for 15 minutes.

5. While the donuts bake, in a shallow bowl, stir together the remaining 2 tablespoons of sugar and 2 teaspoons of cinnamon.

6. Remove the donuts from the oven and brush the tops with the melted butter. Cool the donuts in the pan for 10 minutes, then carefully remove them from the pan and dip the butter-brushed tops in the cinnamon sugar. Transfer to a wire rack to finish cooling.

VARIATION **Mexican Chocolate Donuts:** Add 3 tablespoons of mini chocolate chips to the batter. Instead of dipping in cinnamon sugar, make cinnamon-chocolate glaze by whisking together ¼ cup of confectioners sugar, 1 tablespoon of milk (dairy or plant-based), ½ tablespoon of cocoa powder, ½ tablespoon of butter (or dairy-free butter), ½ teaspoon of ground cinnamon, and ⅛ teaspoon of salt until smooth. Drizzle the glaze over the baked donuts. Allow the glaze to set before serving.

SUBSTITUTION TIPS *You can use 7 tablespoons of granulated sugar in place of the coconut sugar. An equal amount of dairy milk (or another plant-based milk) may be substituted for the unsweetened coconut milk.*

PER SERVING (1 donut): Calories: 202; Total fat: 7g; Total carbs: 34g; Sugar: 14g; Protein: 2g; Fiber: 3g; Sodium: 89mg

FOR THE BATTER

¼ teaspoon coconut oil or avocado oil

190 grams (about 1¼ cups) Gigi's Everyday Gluten-Free Flour (page 27)

60 grams (about ¾ cup) purity protocol oats

½ cup coconut sugar

½ teaspoon salt

½ teaspoon baking powder

¼ teaspoon baking soda

½ cup unsweetened applesauce

1 large egg

¼ cup sunflower oil

2 tablespoons honey

2 teaspoons pure vanilla extract

2 cups zucchini, grated

3 tablespoons chocolate chips

Crumb-Topped Chocolate Chip Zucchini Bread

Vegetarian Chocolate chips on the inside and a layer of sweet crumb topping on top make this zucchini bread dessert-worthy. This recipe is unique for two reasons: First, there's no added liquid because zucchini adds ample moisture. Second, it bakes in a 2-quart dish instead of a loaf or cake pan. I prefer an oval stoneware dish, but any nonmetal 2-quart dish will work.

1. Preheat the oven to 350°F. Grease a 2-quart nonmetal baking dish with the coconut or avocado oil.

2. In a large bowl, combine the flour, oats, sugar, salt, baking powder, and baking soda. Stir to blend.

3. Add the applesauce, egg, sunflower oil, honey, vanilla, zucchini, and chocolate chips. Stir until no dry ingredients remain visible. Spoon the batter into the baking dish.

FOR THE TOPPING

38 grams (about ¼ cup) Gigi's Everyday Gluten-Free Flour (page 27)

20 grams (about ¼ cup) purity protocol oats

2 tablespoons coconut sugar

2 tablespoons dairy-free butter

½ teaspoon ground cinnamon

¼ teaspoon salt

3 tablespoons chocolate chips

4. To make the topping, in a small bowl, stir together the flour, oats, sugar, butter, cinnamon, salt, and chocolate chips until the mixture resembles coarse crumbs. Evenly sprinkle the topping over the batter.

5. Bake for about 40 minutes, or until a toothpick inserted in the center comes out clean. Let cool for 20 minutes before cutting into squares.

VARIATION **Crumb-Topped Apple Cinnamon Bread:** Replace half the zucchini with grated apple, add 1 teaspoon of ground cinnamon to the batter, and omit the chocolate chips. Omit the chocolate chips from the topping and add ¼ teaspoon of ground nutmeg.

PER SERVING Calories: 228; Total fat: 9g; Total carbs: 34g; Sugar: 14g; Protein: 3g; Fiber: 3g; Sodium: 258mg

CHAPTER 14

Naturally Gluten-Free Desserts

The desserts in this chapter are not re-creations of gluten-filled favorites. They are naturally gluten-free and require no extraordinary ingredients like special flour blends or gums. Desserts like these are the best starting points for anyone new to the gluten-free diet. Fruit desserts like Inside-Out Caramel Baked Apples (page 229) and Poached Pears with Butterscotch Sauce (page 226) are recipes that I turned to right after my celiac diagnosis. They helped me realize how many naturally gluten-free foods I already enjoyed. With the recipes in this chapter and throughout the book, you can see how the gluten-free life can be sweeter in so many more ways than you ever imagined!

SERVES 4

Prep time: 15 minutes

Cook time: 40 minutes

FOR THE PEARS

4 cups water

1 cup granulated sugar

4 Bosc pears, peeled

1 lemon, cut into
4 round slices

**FOR THE
BUTTERSCOTCH SAUCE**

¼ cup firmly packed
light brown sugar

¼ cup solid portion
canned coconut milk

2 tablespoons
dairy-free butter

¼ teaspoon salt

1 teaspoon pure
vanilla extract

Coarse sea salt (optional)

Poached Pears with Butterscotch Sauce

Vegan Bosc pears are my favorite variety to use for this dessert because they hold their shape during poaching. If you're new to poaching, it's simply simmering a food in liquid. These pears are easy, elegant, and the results are melt-in-your-mouth delicious. If you eat dairy, this dish is delicious with vanilla ice cream or whipped cream.

1. Place a large saucepan over medium heat and add the water and granulated sugar. Stir to dissolve the sugar.

2. When the sugar is dissolved, completely submerge the pears in the liquid. Tuck the lemon slices around the pears.

3. Bring the liquid to a simmer and cook the pears, uncovered, about 20 minutes, until tender all the way through. To test, carefully pierce the largest part of a pear with a sharp paring knife.

4. Remove the pan from heat and leave the pears in the liquid for 15 minutes. Transfer the pears to a bowl. Discard the poaching liquid and lemon slices.

5. While the pears are soaking off the heat, make the butterscotch sauce. In a medium saucepan over medium-high heat, combine the brown sugar, coconut milk, butter, and salt. Bring to a boil for 4 minutes.

6. Remove from heat and stir in the vanilla. Transfer the sauce to a heat-proof glass container until ready to use. It will thicken as it cools.

7. To serve, place each pear in a dessert bowl and spoon butterscotch sauce over it. Sprinkle a pinch of coarse sea salt on top (if using).

VARIATION **Riesling-Poached Pears:** Replace all the water with an equal amount of Riesling wine.

PER SERVING Calories: 339; Total fat: 16g; Total carbs: 51g; Sugar: 33g; Protein: 2g; Fiber: 7g; Sodium: 192mg

SERVES 14

Prep time: 30 minutes, plus several hours to freeze

5
ING

1 (12-ounce) bag vegan dark chocolate chips

1 tablespoon coconut oil

2 (7-inch) ripe medium bananas

14 ripe strawberries

Frozen Banana Split Stacks

Vegan There are always bananas in at least one of my freezers. Some are mashed, some are sliced, and others are in the form of this better-for-you sweet treat. Kids love these. Because they're so easy to make and relatively healthy, moms don't mind them, either.

1. Line a large baking sheet with wax or parchment paper.

2. In a double boiler, melt the chocolate with the oil just until the chips lose their shape. Alternatively, melt the chocolate and oil in the microwave for 30 seconds on high, stirring every 10 seconds to avoid overheating the chocolate. Stir until smooth.

3. Peel the bananas and cut them crosswise into ½-inch-thick slices. Place the slices on a plate.

4. Wash and dry the strawberries. Hull them and cut them in half. If the berries are very large, slice them into thirds. Place them on a plate.

5. Skewer the fruit on toothpicks, alternating banana slices and strawberry halves until all the fruit is used. You should have about 14 fruited toothpicks, depending on the size of bananas used.

6. Dip the fruited toothpicks into the melted chocolate and place them on the lined baking sheet. Place the pan in the freezer for several hours before serving. To store, transfer the frozen skewers to an airtight container in a single layer and freeze for up to 2 months.

VARIATION 1 **Frozen Stacks Deluxe:** After dipping, top the skewers with chopped nuts, seeds, sprinkles, or coconut, depending on what fits your special diet.

VARIATION 2 **One-Ingredient Ice Cream:** Peel and slice the ripe bananas and freeze until firm. Place the slices in the bowl of a food processor and blend until smooth and creamy. I use 1 medium banana per serving. The riper the bananas are, the sweeter the ice cream will be. Serve in a dessert dish with Frozen Banana Split Stacks on the side.

PER SERVING Calories: 144; Total fat: 8g; Total carbs: 21g; Sugar: 3g; Protein: 2g; Fiber: 1g; Sodium: 0mg

Prep time: 10 minutes

Cook time: 10 minutes

MIN   POT

1 (14-ounce) can full-fat coconut milk

¼ cup pure maple syrup

¼ cup dark cocoa powder

3 tablespoons cornstarch

¼ teaspoon salt

⅓ cup vegan dark chocolate chips

1 tablespoon dairy-free butter

2 teaspoons pure vanilla extract

Vegan Double-Chocolate Pudding

Vegan Thick, creamy, and silky best describes this pudding. Full-fat canned coconut milk lends creaminess, cornstarch adds thickness, and pure maple syrup provides just the right amount of sweetness. I prefer dark cocoa powder and dark chocolate chips for maximum chocolate flavor. Using milk chocolate chips will cause the pudding to be too sweet and bland.

1. Place a 2-quart saucepan over medium-high heat. Put the coconut milk, maple syrup, cocoa powder, cornstarch, and salt in the saucepan. Whisk to combine until the mixture comes to a boil, stirring occasionally. Boil for 30 seconds.

2. Remove the pot from heat and add the chocolate chips, butter, and vanilla. Stir until smooth.

3. Divide the pudding among 4 serving dishes. Let sit at room temperature for 20 minutes before serving.

VARIATION **Mexican Chocolate Pudding:** Add 1 teaspoon of cinnamon and ⅛ teaspoon of cayenne pepper in step 1. Just before serving, top each bowl with dairy-free whipped cream.

SUBSTITUTION TIP *If you eat dairy, use 14 ounces of whole milk and regular chocolate chips and butter.*

PER SERVING Calories: 443; Total fat: 32g; Total carbs: 39g; Sugar: 12g; Protein: 5g; Fiber: 2g; Sodium: 191mg

SERVES 4

Prep time: 10 minutes

Cook time: 40 minutes

4 medium apples,
such as Honeycrisp,
Opal, Empire, Rome, or
Jonathan, cored

4 Medjool dates, pitted

4 teaspoons toasted,
salted pumpkin seeds
(pepitas), divided

4 teaspoons dairy-free
butter, divided

1 teaspoon ground
cinnamon, divided

Inside-Out Caramel Baked Apples

Vegan Caramel and apples go together so well, but traditional caramel is loaded with refined sugar and dairy. In this naturally gluten-free dessert, I use whole-food ingredients to mimic the irresistible caramel-apple flavor. If you're feeling especially indulgent, add a scoop of Three-Ingredient Vegan Vanilla Ice Cream (page 237).

1. Preheat the oven to 375°F.

2. Place the cored apples in an 8-by-8-inch (or similar size) baking dish.

3. Place 1 date in the center of each apple and top each with 1 teaspoon of pumpkin seeds, 1 teaspoon of butter, and ¼ teaspoon of cinnamon.

4. Carefully pour 1 cup of water *around* the apples in the bottom of the pan (not over the apples). Loosely cover with aluminum foil and bake for 20 minutes. Remove the foil and bake for 20 minutes more.

5. Let the apples rest for 15 minutes. Transfer to serving plates and spoon a small amount of the liquid from the pan over the top of each apple. Serve warm.

VARIATION **Sliced Baked Cinnamon Apples:** Cut each cored apple into 8 wedges. Place the wedges in the baking dish and toss with ½ tablespoon of freshly squeezed lemon juice. Add 2 tablespoons of pure maple syrup; 1 tablespoon of cornstarch (optional); 1 tablespoon of melted ghee, butter, or dairy-free butter; 2 teaspoons of ground cinnamon; and a pinch of salt. Omit the dates and pumpkin seeds. Gently stir the apples. Bake at 375°F for 30 minutes, or until tender. Stir and serve as is, over vanilla ice cream, or as a pancake or waffle topping.

PER SERVING Calories: 314; Total fat: 6g; Total carbs: 68g; Sugar: 52g; Protein: 3g; Fiber: 9g; Sodium: 13mg

SERVES 4

Prep time: 20 minutes

Cook time: 50 minutes

4 medium sweet
potatoes

1 tablespoon
sunflower oil

¼ cup pure maple
syrup, divided

2 tablespoons dairy-free
butter, divided

2 tablespoons freshly
squeezed orange juice

¼ teaspoon salt

¼ cup sunflower
seed kernels

1 teaspoon ground
cinnamon

Twice-Baked Sweet Potatoes with Maple-Cinnamon Crunch

Vegan Baking sweet potatoes yields intensified flavor and creamy, buttery flesh. In this recipe, that natural goodness is enhanced with a touch of maple, butter, and orange, then finished with a cinnamon-laced topping that adds a sweet, crunchy texture. This makes a delicious dessert anytime, but my family insists I serve these for Thanksgiving, too! To ensure even baking and portions, choose sweet potatoes similar in size and shape. Depending on the size of potatoes you use, baking time may be affected.

1. Preheat the oven to 400°F. Line a baking sheet with aluminum foil or parchment paper.

2. Wash and dry the potatoes. Place them on the baking sheet and drizzle the oil over them. Rub the oil into each potato. Bake until cooked through, about 40 minutes. Remove the potatoes from the oven, but leave the oven on.

3. When the potatoes are cool enough to handle, split each one lengthwise, scoop out the flesh, and place it in the bowl of a stand mixer. Leave just enough flesh on the peel so that the peel holds together.

4. To the bowl with the sweet potato flesh, add 2 tablespoons of maple syrup, 1 tablespoon of butter, the orange juice, and the salt. Beat until smooth. Spoon the mixture back into the potato skins.

5. In a small bowl, stir together the remaining 2 tablespoons of maple syrup, the remaining 1 tablespoon of butter, the sunflower kernels, and cinnamon. Top the potatoes with this mixture.

6. Bake the potatoes for about 10 minutes, until the sunflower seeds are toasted. Be careful not to overcook the topping, as it can burn easily.

VARIATION **Bourbon Sweet Potatoes with Maple-Cinnamon Crunch:** Omit the orange juice. Add 2 tablespoons of bourbon to the filling.

MAKE-AHEAD TIP *Bake the potatoes up to 3 days ahead. Do not split them. Cool to room temperature and wrap and refrigerate until ready to use. When ready to serve, split the potatoes and prepare the filling. Fill the potatoes and warm in the oven until heated through. Add the topping, then bake for 10 minutes more.*

PER SERVING Calories: 315; Total fat: 13g; Total carbs: 49g; Sugar: 20g; Protein: 4g; Fiber: 5g; Sodium: 235mg

Prep time: 15 minutes, plus 2 hours to chill

COOK ING

1 cup vegan dark chocolate chips

1 can full-fat coconut milk

2 tablespoons pure maple syrup

½ tablespoon pure vanilla extract

⅛ teaspoon salt

Five-Ingredient Chocolate Mousse

Dairy-free · Egg-free · Vegan Canned coconut milk is a magical ingredient. In this recipe, it transforms a handful of ingredients into a rich, creamy chocolate mousse with minimal effort. The high fat content of the canned coconut milk is key. Look for coconut milk with about 14 grams of fat per serving for best results.

1. In a double boiler, melt the chocolate chips until smooth. Remove the double boiler from heat.

2. Spoon the coconut milk—both solid and liquid portions—into a medium mixing bowl and whisk it by hand until smooth, about 30 seconds. Then whisk in the melted chocolate, maple syrup, vanilla, and salt.

3. Pour the mixture into 6 dessert bowls, dividing evenly.

4. Place the bowls in the refrigerator for 2 hours, or until the mousse is set.

PER SERVING Calories: 421; Total fat: 27g; Total carbs: 48g; Sugar: 6g; Protein: 5g; Fiber: 0g; Sodium: 592mg

Prep time: 10 minutes

Cook time: 10 minutes

1 cup sunflower
seed butter

1 cup granulated sugar,
plus more to cross-hatch
the cookies

1 egg, lightly beaten

½ teaspoon pure
vanilla extract

Four-Ingredient Flourless
Not-Peanut-Butter Cookies

Dairy-free • ***Vegetarian*** These are the easiest cookies you'll ever
make. They are naturally gluten-free because no flour is required.
These chewy cookies are traditionally made with peanut butter, but
using sunflower seed butter makes them a delicious nut-free treat
that tastes similar to the original.

1. Preheat the oven to 350°F. Line a baking sheet with parchment paper.

2. In a medium bowl, stir together all the ingredients until smooth.

3. Scoop ½-tablespoon portions onto the baking sheet, spacing them
2 inches apart.

4. Dip a fork in sugar and press the back of the tines into each cookie
to flatten the top slightly. Turn the fork 90 degrees and repeat to make
cross-hatch marks on the cookies.

5. Bake for about 8 minutes, until the edges turn golden and the tops are set.

6. Remove the baking sheet from the oven and let the cookies cool on
the sheet for 2 to 3 minutes before transferring them to a wire rack to
cool completely.

VARIATION 1 **Sweet and Salty Cookies:** Combine 2 tablespoons of sugar and
½ teaspoon of coarse sea salt in a small bowl. Rub the salt between your thumb
and finger to break up any large salt flakes. Stir together and sprinkle over the
cookies before baking.

VARIATION 2 **Chocolate-Drizzled Cookies:** Melt 2 tablespoons of chocolate and
1 teaspoon of coconut oil in a small bowl. Drizzle over the baked, cooled cookies.
Chill briefly to set the chocolate.

ALLERGEN TIP *You can substitute any nut or seed butter that has a similar
consistency to sunflower seed butter or peanut butter.*

PER SERVING Calories: 96; Total fat: 5g; Total carbs: 11g; Sugar: 8g; Protein: 2g; Fiber: 0g; Sodium: 3mg

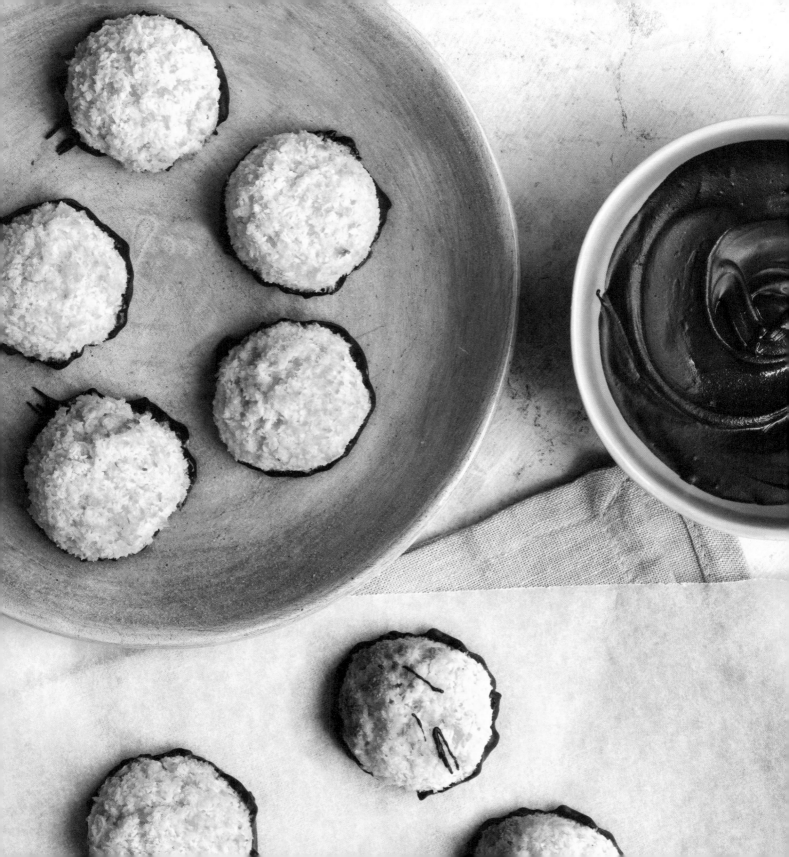

**MAKES 10
(1-TABLESPOON)
MACAROONS**

Prep time: 10 minutes

Cook time: 10 minutes

1 large egg

2½ tablespoons
granulated sugar

1 cup finely shredded
unsweetened coconut

½ teaspoon pure
vanilla extract

2 tablespoons
cornstarch

⅛ teaspoon salt

2 teaspoons orange zest

Orange Essence Macaroons

Dairy-free • ***Vegetarian*** A hint of orange brightens the flavor of these coconut cookies. If you don't need the orange right away after grating the peel, juice it and freeze the juice for another recipe like Grilled Jerk Chicken Tenders (page 167).

1. Preheat the oven to 350°F. Line a baking sheet with parchment paper.

2. In a medium bowl, whisk the egg and sugar together vigorously until frothy, about 2 minutes. Then add the coconut, vanilla, cornstarch, salt, and orange zest. Stir until blended.

3. Scoop level 1-tablespoon measures of batter onto the baking sheet, spacing them a few inches apart.

4. Bake for about 9 minutes, until the macaroons are set and the edges begin to turn golden brown.

5. Remove the baking sheet from the oven and let the macaroons cool completely on the sheet. Store the macaroons in an airtight container for up to 1 week.

VARIATION 1 **Traditional Macaroons:** Omit the orange zest.

VARIATION 2 **Chocolate-Bottom Macaroons:** Melt 3 ounces of dark or semisweet chocolate. When the macaroons are completely cooled, dip the bottoms into the melted chocolate and place the cookies back on the parchment-lined baking sheet. Refrigerate briefly to set the chocolate.

PER SERVING Calories: 154; Total fat: 10g; Total carbs: 14g; Sugar: 9g; Protein: 3g; Fiber: 3g; Sodium: 11mg

FOR THE COATING

1½ cups vegan dark chocolate chips

2 teaspoons coconut oil

FOR THE FILLING

¼ cup sunflower seed butter

1 tablespoon pure maple syrup

½ tablespoon coconut flour

¼ teaspoon salt

Homemade Nut-Free-Butter Cups

Vegan I use organic, single-ingredient sunflower seed butter. If your seed butter contains sugar and salt, omit the maple syrup and salt in this recipe.

1. Line a 12-cup mini muffin tin with parchment liners to prevent sticking. Set aside.

2. To make the coating, place the chocolate chips and oil in a medium microwave-safe bowl. Microwave on high for about 40 seconds, stirring every 10 seconds, until the chocolate is melted. Stir until smooth. Alternatively, melt the chocolate and oil in a double boiler.

3. Into each paper liner, spoon about 2 teaspoons of the melted chocolate coating. Tap the pan to settle the chocolate. Refrigerate the tin for 10 minutes to allow the chocolate to set.

4. While the coating sets, make the filling. In a small bowl, combine the sunflower seed butter, maple syrup, flour, and salt. Stir until smooth and thick. Scoop out 1-teaspoon portions of the filling and form into balls.

5. Remove the muffin tin from the refrigerator. Gently press each ball of filling to flatten it into a disk. Place each disk of filling on top of each chocolate cup.

6. Top each disk of filling with about 1½ teaspoons of melted chocolate. Tap the pan several times to settle the chocolate.

7. Refrigerate for 30 minutes, or until the chocolate is set. Store in an airtight container for up to 2 weeks in the refrigerator.

VARIATION 1 **Almond Butter Cups:** Substitute almond butter for the sunflower seed butter. Omit the coconut flour.

VARIATION 2 **White Chocolate Cups:** If you are not vegan, you can substitute gluten-free white chocolate chips for the dark chocolate.

ALLERGEN TIP *You can use any nut or seed butter that fits your dietary needs.*

PER SERVING Calories: 189; Total fat: 11g; Total carbs: 24g; Sugar: 2g; Protein: 3g; Fiber: 0g; Sodium: 49mg

1 (14-ounce) can full-fat coconut milk, at room temperature

14 ounces unsweetened coconut milk from a carton, chilled

½ cup granulated sugar

3 teaspoons pure vanilla extract

¼ teaspoon salt

Three-Ingredient Vegan Vanilla Ice Cream

Vegan A frozen treat doesn't need to be complicated. With a few ingredients, you can have creamy, dairy-free ice cream in under an hour. I use a countertop ice cream freezer, which yields a delicious soft serve–like consistency in about 40 minutes. For firmer ice cream, I transfer the mixture to the freezer for a couple of hours.

1. In a large bowl, whisk together all the ingredients until well blended.

2. Pour the mixture into an ice cream freezer. Process according to the manufacturer's directions until the ice cream is the consistency of soft serve. For a more solid ice cream, spoon the mixture into a freezer-safe container, cover, and freeze until firm.

VARIATION **Honey-Vanilla Ice Cream:** Honey lends a smoother texture to frozen desserts like this ice cream. Reduce the sugar to ¼ cup and use ¼ cup of honey. The recipe will no longer be vegan, but it will still be dairy-free.

PREPARATION TIP *If the ice cream freezes solid, allow it to sit at room temperature for a few minutes to soften before scooping and serving.*

PER SERVING Calories: 207; Total fat: 14g; Total carbs: 19g; Sugar: 17g; Protein: 2g; Fiber: 0g; Sodium: 169mg

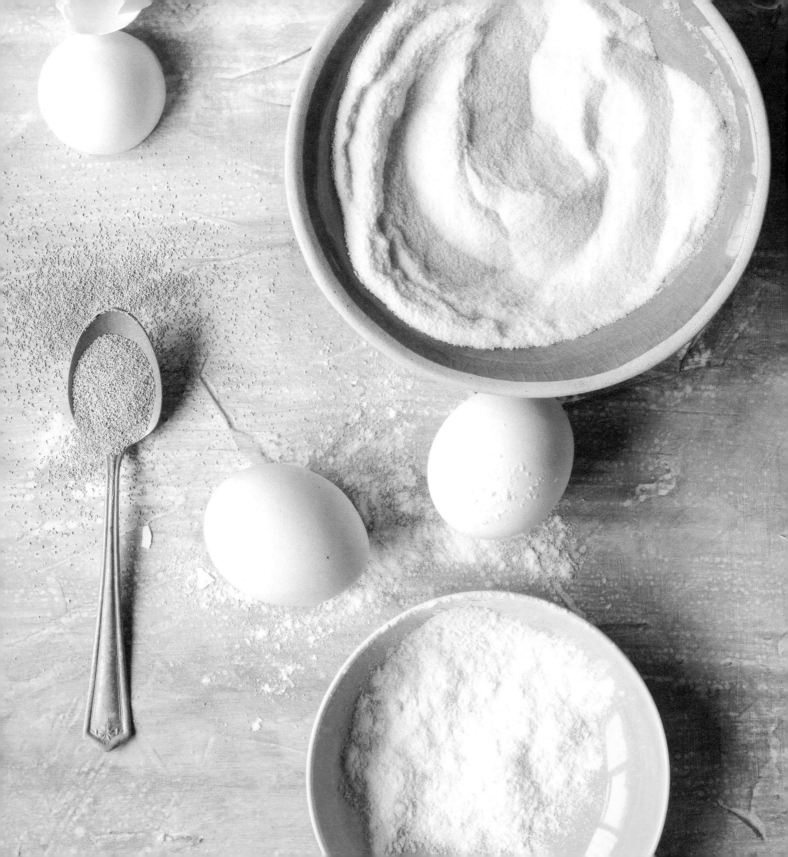

Favorite Gluten-Free Brands

As you embark on your gluten-free journey, you'll discover the products and brands you like best. Here are some of my favorites:

BAKING

- Argo and Rumford brands baking powder (both gluten-free and aluminum-free)
- Arrowhead Mills organic cornmeal
- Equal Exchange baking cocoa and dark chocolate chips
- Fleischmann's fast-acting yeast
- GF Harvest Gluten-Free Rolled Oats
- Glutino pretzels
- Hershey's Special Dark baking cocoa
- Kinnikinnick gluten-free graham-style cracker crumbs
- Madhava organic coconut sugar
- Let's Do . . . Organic unsweetened shredded coconut and coconut flour
- Lily's™ sugar-free chocolate chips
- Wholesome organic confectioners sugar

DAIRY-FREE MILKS

- So Delicious unsweetened coconut milk in a carton
- Native Forest simple organic coconut milk in a can and coconut milk powder

CONDIMENTS, SAUCES, AND SPREADS

- Bragg apple cider vinegar
- Coconut Secret raw coconut aminos
- Dave's Gourmet organic pasta sauce
- Frank's RedHot hot sauce
- Once Again unsalted organic tahini
- Sir Kensington's mayonnaise and Fabanaise (vegan)
- SunButter organic, no-sugar-added sunflower seed butter

FATS AND OILS

- 365 organic sunflower oil
- Earth Balance dairy-free, soy-free buttery spread
- La Tourangelle avocado oil
- Nutiva palm shortening
- Pure Indian Foods ghee
- Vita Coco organic coconut oil

PASTA AND RICE

- Jovial gluten-free pasta
- Lundberg Family Farms organic rices

Special Occasion Menus

KID BIRTHDAY PARTY

- Easy Deli Wraps with Dipping Sauce (page 65)
- Veggie Pizza (page 140)
- Best Yellow Sheet Cake Cupcakes (page 198) with Vegan Cream Cheese Frosting (page 219)

DINNER PARTY

- French Onion Soup (page 108)
- Lemon-Dill Salmon in Parchment (page 154)
- Zesty Roasted Broccoli (page 83)
- Five-Ingredient Chocolate Mousse (page 232)
- Vanilla ice cream

SUPER BOWL SUNDAY

- Gluten-free tortilla chips
- Ultimate Guacamole (page 58)
- Pimiento Cheese Spread (page 61) sandwich on Top 8–Free Sandwich Bread (page 191)
- Easy Pressure Cooker Chili (page 106)
- Four-Ingredient Flourless Not-Peanut-Butter Cookies (page 233)
- Sweet-and-Salty Chocolate Chip Cookies (page 209)

EASTER

- Traditional Deviled Eggs (page 62)
- Apricot & Mustard–Glazed Ham (page 177)
- Yeast-Free Muffin Pan Dinner Rolls (page 186)
- French Carrot Salad (page 72)
- Green Salad with Ranch Dressing (Variation 1, page 33)
- Carrot Cake with Cream Cheese Frosting (page 202)

CHRISTMAS

- Velvety Butternut Squash Soup (page 111)
- Salted Fennel Crackers (page 184)
- Lemon-Herb–Roasted Chicken (Variation 1, page 160)
- Wild Rice Casserole (page 128)
- Roasted Garlic Smashed Cauliflower (page 74)
- Delicate Ginger Cookies (page 207)
- Poached Pears with Butterscotch Sauce (page 226)

Measurement Conversions

VOLUME EQUIVALENTS (LIQUID)

US STANDARD	US STANDARD (OUNCES)	METRIC (APPROXIMATE)
2 tablespoons	1 fl. oz.	30 mL
¼ cup	2 fl. oz.	60 mL
½ cup	4 fl. oz.	120 mL
1 cup	8 fl. oz.	240 mL
1½ cups	12 fl. oz.	355 mL
2 cups or 1 pint	16 fl. oz.	475 mL
4 cups or 1 quart	32 fl. oz.	1 L
1 gallon	128 fl. oz.	4 L

VOLUME EQUIVALENTS (DRY)

US STANDARD	METRIC (APPROXIMATE)
⅛ teaspoon	0.5 mL
¼ teaspoon	1 mL
½ teaspoon	2 mL
¾ teaspoon	4 mL
1 teaspoon	5 mL
1 tablespoon	15 mL
¼ cup	59 mL
⅓ cup	79 mL
½ cup	118 mL
⅔ cup	156 mL
¾ cup	177 mL
1 cup	235 mL
2 cups or 1 pint	475 mL
3 cups	700 mL
4 cups or 1 quart	1 L

OVEN TEMPERATURES

FAHRENHEIT	CELSIUS (APPROXIMATE)
250°F	120°C
300°F	150°C
325°F	165°C
350°F	180°C
375°F	190°C
400°F	200°C
425°F	220°C
450°F	230°C

WEIGHT EQUIVALENTS

US STANDARD	METRIC (APPROXIMATE)
½ ounce	15 g
1 ounce	30 g
2 ounces	60 g
4 ounces	115 g
8 ounces	225 g
12 ounces	340 g
16 ounces or 1 pound	455 g

Recipe Index

	DAIRY-FREE	EGG-FREE	VEGAN	VEGETARIAN
All-American Barbecue Sauce, 32		X		
All-in-One Chicken Tetrazzini, 117	X	X		
All-Vegetable Shepherd's Pie, 138–139	X	X	X	X
Almost-Instant Pressure Cooker Risotto, 125	X	X	X	X
Apricot & Mustard–Glazed Ham, 177	X	X		
Avocado Toast, 59	X	X	X	X
Baked Cinnamon Sugar Donuts, 220–221	X			X
Barbecue Chicken Pizza, 169		X		
Barbecue Chicken Salad Bowl, 86	X			
Belgian Waffles, 42				X
Best Yellow Sheet Cake, 198	X			X
BLT Bow Tie Pasta Salad, 114	X			
Blueberry Coffee Cake, 206	X			X
Breakfast Burritos, 55	X			X
Breakfast Casserole, 54				
Brussels & Butternut Bowl with Crispy Bacon, 87	X	X		
Caprese Quesadilla, 66		X		X
Carrot Cake with Cream Cheese Frosting, 202–203				X
Cheddar & Chive Muffins, 193				X
Cheeseburger Lovers' Salad, 88	X			
Cheesy Hummus-Filled Manicotti, 120		X		X
Chicken Fajitas, 165	X	X		
Chicken Pot Pie, 162	X	X		
Chicken Tamale Pie, 168	X			
Chimichurri Salmon Salad, 89	X	X		
Chocolate Chip Oatmeal Cookies, 210	X			X

	DAIRY-FREE	EGG-FREE	VEGAN	VEGETARIAN
Chocolate Kentucky Bourbon Pie, 214				X
Cilantro-Lime Slaw, 73	X	X	X	X
Classic Brownies, 217	X			X
Classic French Toast, 43				X
Classic Scones, 48	X			X
Cobb Salad with Strawberry Vinaigrette, 90	X			
Cod with Lemon-Caper Sauce, 157	X	X		
Corn-Avocado Salsa, 77	X	X	X	X
Cornbread, 189	X			X
Creamy Chilled Green Soup, 101	X	X	X	X
Creamy Dairy-Free Mushroom Soup, 104	X	X	X	X
Creamy Spinach with Cardamom, 79		X		X
Creamy Tomato Soup, 103	X	X	X	X
Crispy Chicken Strips, 164	X			
Crispy Oven Fries, 80	X	X	X	X
Crispy Skillet Fish Cakes, 156	X			
Crumb-Topped Chocolate Chip Zucchini Bread, 222–223				X
Deconstructed Potato Salad Bowl, 93	X			
Delicate Ginger Cookies, 207	X			X
Double-Crust Apple Pie, 212–213	X			X
Easy Brazilian Rolls, 187				X
Easy Deli Wraps with Dipping Sauce, 65	X			
Easy Flank Steak, 175	X	X		
Easy Lo Mein, 129	X	X		X
Easy Pressure Cooker Chili, 106	X	X		
Farmers' Market Pasta Skillet, 123		X		X
Five-Ingredient Chocolate Mousse, 232	X	X	X	X
Five-Ingredient No-Sugar Granola Bars, 68–69		X		X
Five-Minute Pizza/Pasta Sauce, 31	X	X	X	X

	DAIRY-FREE	EGG-FREE	VEGAN	VEGETARIAN
Mini Meatloaves, 171	X			
Mock Chicken Salad, 141	X	X	X	X
Mushroom, Potato & Zucchini Enchiladas, 144		X		X
New York–Style Cheesecake, 204–205				X
No-Boil Pasta Bake, 116				X
Nutritious Double-Chocolate Bites, 67	X	X	X	
One-Bowl Chocolate Cake, 200–201	X			X
The Only Pie Crust You'll Ever Need, 37	X	X	X	X
Orange Essence Macaroons, 235	X			X
Parmesan Polenta, 132		X		X
Pasta with Chicken in Ratatouille-Style Sauce, 121	X	X		
Pasta with Tilapia Matecumbe, 119	X	X		
Perfect Gravy Every Time, 35	X	X		
Perfect Scrambled Eggs, 50				X
Persian-Spiced Carrot Hummus, 60	X	X	X	X
Persian-Spiced Spaghetti Squash Bake, 146	X			X
Pimiento Cheese Spread, 61				X
Pizza Crust, 29–30	X	X	X	X
Poached Pears with Butterscotch Sauce, 226	X	X	X	X
Pressure Cooker Cuban Black Bean Soup, 105	X	X	X	X
Pressure Cooker Lamb Stew, 98	X	X		
Pressure Cooker Red Lentil Soup, 99	X	X	X	X
Pressure Cooker Spiced Short Ribs, 173	X	X		
Pressure Cooker Spicy Cream of Cauliflower Soup, 107	X	X	X	X
Pressure Cooker Vegan Mac 'n Cheese, 115	X	X	X	X
Quick & Easy Banana Bread, 46	X			X
Quick Baking Mix, 26	X	X	X	X
Roasted Garlic Smashed Cauliflower, 74–75	X	X		
Roasted Harissa Chicken, 160	X	X		

	DAIRY-FREE	EGG-FREE	VEGAN	VEGETARIAN
Roasted Lemon Chicken with Potatoes, 163	X	X		
Salted Fennel Crackers, 184–185	X	X	X	X
Savory Baked Oatmeal, 134	X			
Sheet Pan Eggs in Sweet Potato Nests, 52	X			X
Sheet Pan Shrimp with Shortcut Remoulade, 152	X			
Sheet Pan Tilapia with Ginger-Lime Butter, 155	X	X		
Slow Cooker Barbecue Pork, 178		X		
Slow Cooker Garden Vegetable Soup, 100	X	X	X	X
Slow Cooker Korean Beef Roast, 176	X	X		
Slow Cooker Luck & Money, 110	X	X	X	X
Smoked Salmon Roll-Ups, 64		X		
Sour Cream Coconut Cake, 199				X
Sour Cream Dinner Rolls, 188		X		X
Southern Corn Pudding, 78	X			X
Southern-Style Panzanella, 95	X			X
Speedy Beef Stroganoff, 172	X			
Spicy Southern-Style Shrimp, 153	X	X		
Spinach, Artichoke & Quinoa–Stuffed Peppers, 133				X
Strawberry Crumble, 211	X	X	X	X
Stuffed Pork Chops with Cumin & Fresh Herbs, 180–181	X	X		
Sunflower Seed Butter Muffins, 49	X	X	X	X
Superfood Salad, 92	X	X		
Sweet Potato Fritters, 82	X			X
Sweet Potato Sausage Balls, 179	X	X		
Sweet-and-Salty Chocolate Chip Cookies, 209	X	X	X	X
Sweet-and-Spicy Ruby-Glazed Drumsticks, 161	X	X		
Tex-Mex Stuffed Sweet Potatoes, 147	X	X	X	X
Three-Ingredient Key Lime Parfait, 215	X	X	X	X
Three-Ingredient Vegan Vanilla Ice Cream, 237	X	X	X	X

	DAIRY-FREE	EGG-FREE	VEGAN	VEGETARIAN
Tomato Quiche with Goat Cheese & Avocado, 148–149				X
Top 8–Free Sandwich Bread, 191–192	X	X	X	X
Traditional Deviled Eggs, 62	X			X
Traditional Meatballs, 170	X	X		
Turmeric-Honey Baked Chicken Breasts, 166	X	X		
Twice-Baked Sweet Potatoes with Maple-Cinnamon Crunch, 230–231	X	X	X	X
Ultimate Guacamole, 58	X	X	X	X
Vegan Cream Cheese Frosting, 219	X	X	X	X
Vegan Double-Chocolate Pudding, 228	X	X	X	X
Vegan Tikka Masala, 145	X	X	X	X
Vegetable Fried Rice, 135	X	X	X	X
Veggie Pizza, 140		X		X
Velvety Butternut Squash Soup, 111	X	X	X	X
Versatile Flatbread, 194–195	X			X
Wild Rice Casserole, 128	X	X	X	X
Yeast-Free Muffin Pan Dinner Rolls, 186	X			X
Zesty Roasted Broccoli, 83	X	X	X	X
Zucchini & Pasta with Creamy Herb Sauce, 124	X	X	X	X

Index

About the Author

GIGI STEWART, BS, MA, is the creator of the popular lifestyle website GigiStewart.com. Having lived with chronic pain for 25 years, Gigi pursued a career in inflammatory pain research to find answers. In 2007, her health took a nosedive. A diagnosis of celiac disease exposed the cause of her poor health, including a series of strokes that nearly claimed her life.

With a new lease on life, the spirited Southern belle put her research skills to work to learn how to heal her shattered immune system with a gluten-free diet. Gigi took her science to the kitchen to create gluten-free versions of family-favorite recipes. When friends and family couldn't tell them from the "real thing," her Southern gentleman encouraged her to share them "to save others from going through what you did."

In 2009, Gigi traded her crisp lab coat for a frilly apron and claimed her spot online, sharing original recipes and her signature Smart Nutrition Backed by Science. Gigi's fact-based approach, positive attitude, and compassionate nature earned her the trust of a broad audience.

In 2018, Gigi revamped and expanded her website to offer readers more, because above all else, it is her genuine desire to help others live their best lives.